Praise for *An Anthology of Canadian Birth Stories*

"This book is a 'must-read' for expectant parents, because it will help them to make the right birthing choices for themselves, and for those who have already given birth, because it will help them to better understand their own birthing experiences.

This book makes a great contribution to the field of reproductive studies, and an even greater contribution to child bearers and birthgivers, because it provides its readers with a plethora of exquisitely written birth stories. These stories cover the gamut of possible childbirth experiences, from marvelous home births to wonderful and not-so-wonderful hospital births. The overall messages that come through loud and clear are that *birth matters*, both to birthgivers and to their families, and that child bearers' voices must be heard and heeded."

—**Robbie Davis-Floyd** (PhD), world-renowned scholar on birth and author of *Birth as an American Rite of Passage* and of *Ways of Knowing about Birth: Mothers, Midwives, Medicine, and Birth Activism*

"The stories cover births of all kinds: rapid, unmedicated, epiduralized, surgical, preterm birth, preeclampsia and stillbirth, and all kinds of perinatal providers: doulas, midwives, nurses, and physicians. All are described with respect and positive energy. Coping with labor is not instinctive. Humans require support. Each generation needs to learn how to give this support. The writers in *An Anthology* pass on the instructions for labor coping in their stories without being dogmatic. Those who read this book while expecting will have many visions of labor and birth to drawn on."

—**Cecilia M. Jevitt** (RM, CNM, APRN, PhD, FACNM), Director of Midwifery and Associate Professor in the Department of Family Practice in the Faculty of Medicine at University of British Columbia

"This book is a much needed book! *An Anthology of Canadian Birth Stories* is a wonderful read. Whether you want stories of empowering births, both home and hospital, or are looking for information on birth justice and the rights of childbearing families, this book is for you. The authors shared their stories with vulnerability which was inspiring! There is so much to learn from these stories and information following. Also includes info about birth Justice, rights of childbearing families, and clarifies the role of the doula. My take home: You have a voice and your voice deserves to be heard."

—**Jenn Fountaine** (LCCE, CD/BDT(DONA), PCD(DONA), CLE, FACCE), DONA International Birth Doula Training, Lamaze Program Director, and Birth and Postpartum Doula

"This anthology is a must read of firsthand experiences and insightful wisdom for birthing families and those that support them. There is a powerful impact in hearing firsthand the joys and struggles of birthing families. This anthology will have you laughing, crying and ready to jump in and take action!"

—**Sondra Marcon**, Education Director and Instructor, Doula Training Canada, Association of Ontario Doulas' board member

"*An Anthology of Canadian Birth Stories* is a MUST READ for every new doula. The book takes you through a journey of just how varied birth experiences can be. It reinforces that satisfaction with birth has EVERYTHING to do with how we're supported, not just the outcome we had hoped for. The book will bring you through every emotion and inspire you to continue your work as a birth worker, reinforcing the DEEP INNER KNOWING that we are needed more than ever before."

—**Stefanie Antunes** (LCCE, FACCE, BDT/CD/PCD(DONA), Association of Ontario Doulas' board member, Founder of Doula School

"The art of storytelling has the power to bring people together, transform and heal. This enriching book does all these things, and so much more. You will laugh, you will cry and will open you up to the myriad of experiences that pregnancy brings. This book is for anyone who wants to celebrate and revel in the human experience of birth and consider ways we can better support birthing families."

—**Sarah Chisholm**, Registered Midwife with Community Midwives of Kingston.

"As a birth doula trainer and advocate, I believe that it's essential to continue to share positive birth stories to promote pleasure and less fear-based birth. The book serves as an excellent resource for anyone interested in learning about childbirth from a diverse range of experiences and perspectives. Thank you Laura Pascoe & Josée Leduc for putting such an inspiring Anthology together!"

—**Debra Pascali-Bonaro**, (B.Ed., LCCE, PDT/BDT(DONA))

Praeclarus Press, LLC
2504 Sweetgum Lane
Amarillo, Texas 79124 USA
806-367-9950
www.PraeclarusPress.com

All rights reserved. No part of this publication may be reproduced or transmitted in any form, or by any means, electronic or mechanical, including photocopy, recording, stored in a database, or any information storage, or put into a computer, without the prior written permission from the publisher.

DISCLAIMER: The information contained in this publication is advisory only and is not intended to replace sound clinical judgment or individualized patient care. The author disclaims all warranties, whether expressed or implied, including any warranty as the quality, accuracy, safety, or suitability of this information for any particular purpose.

ISBN: 978-1-946665-59-1

Cover Design: Ken Tackett
Copyediting: Chris Tackett
Layout & Design: Nelly Murariu
Copyright © 2023 Laura Pascoe & Josée Leduc
Copyright © 2020 by Ashley Lightfoot for *Birth of the Tiger*
Copyright © 2019 by Mandee MacDonald for *A Blazing Birth*
Copyright © 2020 by Lori Sebastianutti for *Cutting Ties and Letting Go*
Copyright © 2019 by Karen Price for *A Healing Birth*
Copyright © 2020 by Mercedes Papalia for *Luna Rising*
Copyright © 2019 by Janelle Connor for *Riding a Tsunami*
Copyright © 2020 by Camille Ramsberger for *It all Makes Sense Now*
Copyright © 2020 by Angela Douglas for *Worth it*
Copyright © 2020 by Brittany Oliver for *Birth Plan*
Copyright © 2020 by Christine Folan for *Delivered*
Copyright © 2020 by Leah Timmerman for *She Who Brings Forth the Blossoms*
Copyright © 2020 by Dana MacDonald for *Our Rainbow*
Copyright © 2020 by Jenna Kovacic for *Believing in your Body*
Copyright © 2020 by Danielle BoByk for *Reclaiming My Birth Story*
Copyright © 2020 by Julie Meier for *Mother Knows Best*
Copyright © 2020 by Kristin Nuttall for *A Full Moon Eclipse Birth*
Copyright © 2020 by Alison Ryder for *Just Like Hollywood*
Copyright © 2020 by Sharon Chisvin for *Labour, Delivery and a Grateful Grandmother*
Copyright © 2020 by Sara Wettlaufer for *A Dramatic Debut*
Copyright © 2019 by Mica Pants for *The Dark Road to Life*
Copyright © 2020 by Sheena McDonald for *Surprise!*
Copyright © 2020 by Sara Wood-Gates for *Wednesday's Child*
Copyright © 2019 by Gretchen Huntley for *The Middle Child*
Copyright © 2019 by Anne-Marie Laplante for *Oliver's Birth*
Copyright © 2019 by Scarlete Flores-Singh for *In Gratitude*
Copyright © 2019 by Rebecca Young for *A Doula Letter*
Copyright © 2019 by Bonnie Jean-Louis for *My Mom Job Journey*
Copyright © 2020 by Sabrina Malach for *Curbside Delivery*
Copyright © 2020 by Jennifer Osmond for *After Hours*
Copyright © 2020 by Lisa Brenner for *At Light Speed*
Copyright © 2020 by Aly Guildford for *Miles to Journey Through*
Copyright © 2020 by Jessica Cheyne for *Through the Doulas' Eyes*

Our deepest gratitude to all the writers who generously gave us permission to publish their birth stories, and to those who contributed to the book without any monetary compensation. All proceeds from the sale of this book go to the Doula Support Foundation to provide high quality and inclusive doula care to Canadian low-income families.

An Anthology of Canadian Birth Stories

*Inspiration and Essential Guidance
for Parents, Parents-to-be, and
Healthcare Providers*

Edited by Laura Pascoe & Josée Leduc

Praeclarus Press. LLC
©2023. The Doula Support Foundation. All rights reserved
www.PraeclarusPress.com

CONTENTS

Author's Note	9
Foreword	11
Introduction	19
The Doula Support Foundation: A Short Story of our Birth	25

Birth Stories — 29

Birth of the Tiger by Ashley Lightfoot	31
A Blazing Birth by Mandee MacDonald	41
Cutting Ties and Letting Go by Lori Sebastianutti	47
A Healing Birth by Karen Price	55
Luna Rising by Mercedes Papalia	61
Riding a Tsunami by Janelle Connor	69
It All Makes Sense Now by Camille Ramsperger	79
Worth It by Angela Douglas	87
Birth Plan by Brittany Oliver	93
Delivered by Christine Folan	97
She Who Brings Forth the Blossoms by Leah Timmermann	105
Our Rainbow by Dana MacDonald	113
Reclaiming My Birth Story by Danielle BoByk	117
Believing in Your Body by Jenna Kovacic	121
Mother Knows Best by Julie Meier	127
A Full Moon Eclipse Birth by Kristin Nuttall	131
Through the Doula's Eyes: A Photo Story by Jessica Cheyne	137
Just Like Hollywood by Alison Ryder	145
A Dramatic Debut by Sara Wettlaufer	151
Surprise! by Sheena McDonald	155
Wednesday's Child by Sara Wood-Gates	161
Labour, Delivery, and a Grateful Grandmother by Sharon Chisvin	167
The Dark Road to Life by Mica Pants	173
The Middle Child by Gretchen Huntley	179
Oliver's Birth by Anne-Marie Laplante	183

In Gratitude by Scarlete Flores-Singh	187
A Doula Letter by Carrie Allen	191
My Mom Job Journey by Bonnie Jean-Louis	197
Curbside Delivery by Sabrina Malach	203
After Hours by Jennifer Osmond	207
At Light Speed by Lisa Brenner	213
Miles to Journey Through by Aly Guildford	219

Birth Sharing Circles: Hosting Your Own — 225

Essential Evidence-Based Guidance for Birth — 229

What is a Doula and How Can They Help Me? by Laura Pascoe	230
Choosing a Healthcare Provider and the Birth Setting by Laura Pascoe and Josée Leduc	237
Indigenous Birthing and Canada's Birth Evacuation Policy by Karen Lawford	249
Birthing as a Racialized Person: What Everyone Should Know by Chandra Martini	253
Perinatal Care and Human Rights by Lauren Miller	260
Supporting Success: How Birthing Practices May Affect Breastfeeding by Dr. Jack Newman and Teresa Pitman of the International Breastfeeding Centre	265
Recipe for a Satisfying Birth by Josée Leduc	271
International Childbirth Initiative: 12 Steps to Safe and Respectful MotherBaby-Family Maternity Care	275

Contributors, Contest's Jurors, and Artists	279
Reading List	289
Acknowledgements	291
References	295

AUTHOR'S NOTE

For many women, pregnancy and childbirth are experiences that meaningfully and powerfully connect them to a sense of womanhood, the exquisitely feminine, and solidarity with other women. This is a beautiful thing. And, there are many others who do not identify as women who also become pregnant and give birth. These individuals equally deserve a sense of empowerment and solidarity in their experience. Most research on pregnancy and childbirth uses the terms "women" and "mother"—and these are appropriate, even empowering terms for many throughout their birthing journeys. Having a gendered lens to understand where and how misogyny shows up in the institutions surrounding childbirth is also critically important. And, the experiences and needs of those who do not identify neatly within the "woman" box—gender non-conforming people, transgender folks—are equally as important, as are efforts to ensure these individuals are seen, heard, cared for, and respected along their reproductive journeys.

Our hope for this book is that it contributes to a positive and empowering culture around birth *for everyone who births and/or experiences pregnancy loss.* As such, we have used terms such as "birthgiver" and "pregnant person" where possible. For the birth stories, we left each writer's preferred terminology. Where research and data specifically use the terms "women" and/or "mother" and we deem it inaccurate to change to a more gender inclusive term (because the data only represent those who identify as women), we reflect the terms used in the original studies.

FOREWORD
by Michael C. Klein

Homage to Dr. Murray Enkin and the Complexity of Evidence-Based Medicine

Murray Enkin was a pioneer in Family-Centred Maternity Care in the 1960s and 70s, during a time when partners were excluded from birth and the decision-making around non-evidence-based procedures like routine episiotomy, shaving, intravenous drips, enemas, routine induction, and ubiquitous electronic fetal monitoring (some of which, unfortunately, remain the norm). My dear friend and mentor died at age 97 on June 6th, 2021. For me and the birth community, it was a huge loss, both because of who he was and what he represented. As an almost retired family physician and family medicine professor, greatly inspired by Murray's prescience and brilliance, I'd like to share reflections on Murray's influence on me and generations of women.

Starting out as a general practitioner, Murray soon reinvented himself—the first of several reinventions—when he retrained as an obstetrician. Murray questioned everything, including his own ideas about what was normal. Often a curmudgeon, he was ready to heartily and critically engage with practices, authority, his colleagues, and politicians. A Jewish man heading a department of obstetrics and gynecology in a Catholic hospital, he set out to question what was considered routine. What was the evidence? Why do we do this? Who started this nonsense? How do we change it?

Undoubtedly influenced by the death in childbirth of his grandmother and witnessing dehumanized care for women when in medical school, he found himself unable to accept how women were treated. He and his wife Eleanor were dedicated to listening and seeking to understand women and their labour and birth experiences—negative or positive. Murray and Eleanor had a special partnership, often visiting with labouring women together, with Eleanor taking magnificent birth photos to share with women and their partners.

When McMaster Medical School was founded, Murray left private practice to be one of the first faculty members, beginning a path that engaged him with many of today's leaders and all types of maternity care providers. Embarrassed to learn that obstetrics was the least evidence-based speciality, he joined the movement to make obstetrics evidence-based. With colleagues at the National Perinatal Epidemiology Unit in Oxford, they set out to question all procedures and approaches used in caring for pregnant and labouring women. In so doing, they developed the Oxford Database of Perinatal Trials, systematically studying all the taken-for-granted beliefs about what was needed or not, what was useful, and what was harmful.

In those heady days of the 1970s and 1980s, Murray became one of the principal spokespersons for the randomized controlled trial (RCT) as the only serious way of knowing, culminating in the massive two-volume book: *Effective Care in Pregnancy and Childbirth* (Enkin, Kierse, & Chalmers, 1989). This quickly became the Bible for the field and counted as the main force in the development of evidence-based medicine (EBM) throughout medicine—not just obstetrics. I will be forever grateful to Murray for encouraging me to do an RCT of episiotomy in Canada. Why in Canada? Because several excellent midwifery-run RCTs of episiotomy had been done in Europe and beyond—all showing benefits to limiting episiotomy only to specific indications—and it was time to systematically examine this practice on our home turf.

North American obstetricians ordinarily did not read midwifery literature, and if they had, they would have dismissed it as irrelevant to physician practice. So, following Murray's recommendation, I designed a study of physicians caring for more than 1000 women in normal university and community hospital practice in Montreal. Recognizing that physicians would be more likely to accept the results if the study included additional "scientific" measures, I developed and included never-before-used measurements of pelvic floor functioning before and after labour. We employed electromyographic perineometry, which, in lay language, is "kegelometry." The study clearly showed that routine episiotomy caused the very vaginal and pelvic floor trauma that it was supposed to prevent (Klein et al., 1994; Klein et al., 1995; Klein et al., 1997). One example is that 52 of 53 severe vaginal traumas in the trial occurred in the presence of episiotomy—and only one without episiotomy.

The evidence spoke for itself; routine episiotomy did far more damage than good. Encouragingly, these findings were accepted in North America, and the section in obstetrical textbooks on episiotomy had to be completely rewritten. Over the next 10 years, episiotomy rates in North America dropped from at least 65-70 percent to 12 percent, and severe trauma rates dropped from 4.5 percent to 1.5 percent. This saved, and continues to save, many women from unnecessary birth trauma. But even today there are holdouts and pushback based on questionable research. (The struggles to get funded and published for an RCT that challenged conventional wisdom is detailed in my book *Dissident Doctor: Catching Babies and Challenging the Medical Status Quo* (Klein, 2018).) This study of episiotomy became the start for virtually all my subsequent research. Without Murray's influence, none of this would have happened.

Even as evidence-based medicine was becoming accepted, Murray himself began to question RCTs as the only way of knowing (Enkin et al., 2006). He pointed out that the RCT was ideal for studying *complicated* issues but not *complex* ones. RCTs work for simple problems like comparing drug A with drug B but not for complex issues involving human behaviour and beliefs, practice settings, and practitioner skill sets. Episiotomy might appear to be simple or only somewhat complicated, but because of entrenched beliefs about episiotomy, many RCT study doctors had great difficulty following the trial protocol (Klein, 1995).

Murray was an early promoter of the re-emergence of regulated midwifery, doulas, and home birth with trained integrated midwifery. His arguments and history were so respected that his voice could not be ignored. His students heard him, and many followed his lead. However, he once told me that he regretted getting involved with RCTs. Perhaps overstated, this is because he understood that even RCTs could be distorted and misused. He developed what some of us call "Enkins First Law": "The RCT is perfectly designed to show the results for the conditions under which the RCT is conducted—BUT only for those conditions." For example, suppose the RCT is conducted in a university hospital where only obstetricians and hospital-based nurses practice, and the background caesarean section rate is, let's say, 12-15 percent. In that case, the study has relevance (internal validity) for such settings and practices. But that result may not be relevant or applicable (external validity) for community or midwifery practice, or in settings with much higher cesarean section rates that are today's norm.

Murray clearly understood that politically motivated and biased RCTs could be designed in advance to produce the desired results. This concept was best stated by the late obstetrician Philip Hall, who said, "We have moved from evidence-based decision-making to decision-based evidence-making." (Klein 2009).

In the spirit of this book, I have included a story from *Dissident Doctor:*

Making Trouble in Vancouver

Several years before leaving Montreal for a new position in Vancouver in 1993, I was invited to Vancouver to give a talk. I spoke about some of my research and how it can impact practice and lead to changes in practice. The audience specifically wanted to hear about the RCT of episiotomy. Later that day there was a panel on birth. The panelists were a lawyer, an obstetrician, a family doctor (me), and a woman (billed as "the consumer"). She was the first to speak, and told of her first birth, which she thought was horrible. She stated that her wishes and needs were ignored and the birth was, in her opinion, unnecessarily traumatic. She described her second birth with a family physician colleague as wonderful. Her wishes were respected, and she felt that her needs were discussed and implemented.

At the end of her presentation, a very angry obstetrician in the audience attacked her as being interested only in *herself* and *her* experience. He stated that she did not care about the health of her newborn. He said that what she had done was tantamount to child abuse. The audience was shocked, hushed. I was due to talk next. I had prepared a detailed written contribution. Instead of giving my talk I said, "Now you can see why women are having home births—anything to keep out of the clutches of a practitioner like this." And I sat down. The audience went wild. Half supported me. The other half felt that I was rude and disrespectful. This event coloured the rest of the conference, with various proponents of different approaches to birth arguing among themselves and with me.

Two days later, my host drove me to the airport for my return to Montreal, still talking about the event. We were in the coffee shop when I noticed Margaret Atwood sitting at another table. I pointed her out to my host, who became excited and asked if I knew her. I explained that I had met her when my wife Bonnie was making the film, *Not a Love Story*. I said that she probably wouldn't remember me, and she looked tired and engaged. Under continued pressure, I finally agreed to say hello. She was friendly and invited us to sit with her. She immediately began, in her role as a curious reporter/novelist, to ask what I was doing in Vancouver. I told her that I had given a talk. She wanted to know more detail, so I told her the story about the panel. After a pause she said: "I think you've got it wrong. It is you doctors who are the consumers! It is we women who are the providers."

I only later learned that she was on a book tour for her just-published *The Handmaid's Tale*. When I later read the novel, I fully understood her interest in my story. The book describes a dystopia when women are merely vessels for producing babies for the state. They have no rights, and their children are taken away to be given to "more worthy" childless recipients. I think of Atwood's words when I see or hear of a birth that is fully "managed," real "birth control," where the woman is ignored, and her contributions are dismissed. I hoped that Atwood's look into the future would not happen.

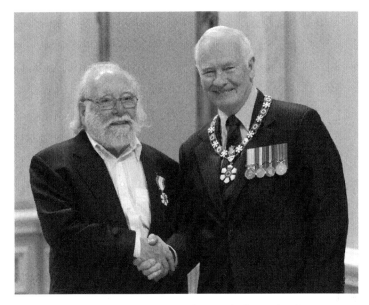

Murray receiving the Order of Canada from the Governor General for his efforts on behalf of the women of Canada.

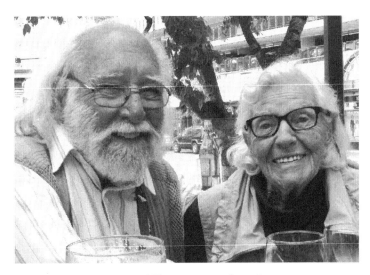

Murray and Eleanor, together always.

There has been some progress, but that type of experience, sadly, is not rare. Since the 2016 Trump election and U. S. Supreme Court ruling on abortion, the reissued *The Handmaid's Tale* is more chilling and relevant than ever.

So how can pregnant women navigate the dance between evidence-based medicine and their hoped-for birth? Asking their chosen provider specific questions will help determine if and how the provider's values align with the views and practices of the birthing person. Here are some suggested questions from my years of supporting women's births:

- What routines are employed in your practice?
- Do your team/partners/coverage groups share that approach? If not, how does it differ?
- What are your attitudes toward routine episiotomy and induction in pregnancies that go past due dates?

Discussions of these questions will give the pregnant person an idea of the provider's birth philosophy and, hopefully, shared values. That the practitioner employs high quality evidence-based medicine is important, but this must be situated in the context of what is important to the woman (and her partner). This dialogue between the patient and the practitioner should result in a trusting relationship that is grounded on helping the patient make evidence-informed decisions that are right for her and her family. Both Murray and I were committed to a shared, reciprocal, patient-professional relationship long before the era of Birth Plans (Klein, 1983). If the provider says something like, "Don't worry. I will do what is necessary. Leave it to me," it's time to change providers.

Each woman planning a birth brings a unique and complex set of values and circumstances that can be informed, enlightened, and guided by evidence and then integrated into her approach to her birth as she negotiates her plan with her providers. Early in Murray's evolution, he clearly articulated the importance of women's beliefs, experiences, and stories as fundamental to the appreciation of birth and essential to the next revolution in childbirth. The success of Family-Centred Childbirth in the 1970s was just the first step in a process. It was driven by women and not professionals. The next step in changing an overmedicalized, industrialized, and infantized childbirth healthcare system will also have to be driven by women. It is my hope that the narratives in this book will help to show many ways forward.

Michael C Klein CM, MD, FCFP CCFP FAAP (neonatal-perinatal)
Emeritus Professor
Family Practice & Pediatrics
University of British Columbia
Sr. Scientist Emeritus
BC Children's Hospital Research Institute, Vancouver
mklein@mail.ubc.ca
www.michaelcklein.ca
Author of *Dissident Doctor: Catching Babies and Challenging the Medical Status Quo*

To learn more about Dr. Murray Enkin: *Enjoying the Interval: Murray Enkin: A Life Medical Humanist and Honorary Midwife* by Kerreen M. Reiger

INTRODUCTION

As birth doulas, we have the great fortune to listen to many birth stories. It is often the first thing clients want to share if they have previously birthed. Whether clients or other dear ones, we often see birthgivers with a need to process their childbirth experiences, even years later. For many, the eagerness to share is mixed with trepidation, as though they are not used to fully sharing their story; as though giving birth is not a story needing to be told, reflected on, and held with respect and awe. Writing one's own birth story is a way to process, as is reading the stories of others. Birth stories have the capacity to inspire, empower, and even heal. That is the beauty of sharing stories.

Even beyond birth, storytelling has been used to pass on culture, knowledge, and beliefs for thousands of years. Storytelling is a fundamental human instinct, and even our *memory* is story-based. Stories shape our memories, how we recall events as well as how we perceive the world around us. Storytelling evokes emotional responses and cultivates connection with one another. Stories have the power to influence, teach, and motivate people.

Why is storytelling such a powerful mode of communication? In conveying information through story, experience is endowed with meaning, and research shows that storytelling fosters connection and builds empathy. As 20th century German philosopher Walter Benjamin argued, while the outcome of analytic thinking is *information,* the product of storytelling is *wisdom.* Put simply, storytelling has the incredible capacity to transform *information* into *wisdom.*

Storytelling around birth has drastically changed over the last few generations. The medicalization of childbirth[1] has meant that birth stories have

---

[1] When we say, "medicalization of childbirth," we are referring to the ways that, starting in the 17th century, birth became an increasingly enticing—and lucrative—area for the emerging medical field to occupy. This included a push to birth in hospitals instead of at home, attendance by male physicians and later obstetricians instead of midwives (which was linked to the move to hospitals, where midwives were barred from providing services), and a reliance on pharmaceutical pain relief and medical intervention to manage the birthing process.

increasingly been left untold, and those who birth are increasingly unfamiliar with the birthing process. Fear has replaced a sense of control and ownership over birth for many people, and the community that is built around sharing birth wisdom and knowledge has been ruptured and weakened.

This is why telling birth stories, *writing* birth stories, is so important. Birth stories help to redirect our focus back to birthing people's preferences and their active and essential role in decision-making. Birth stories rightfully place the birthing person at the centre of the birthing event, rather than rendering them a passive participant. As perinatal nurse and scholar Jane Staton Savage once wrote, "When positive birth stories are shared, special messages are conveyed that describe the courage and power of women as birthgivers, the integrity of the birth process, and the sanctity of the family … These stories have the potential to change the beliefs of those who become vicarious learners" (2001, p. 4).

In 2019 the Doula Support Foundation began an annual Birth Story Writing Contest. This book is a compilation of the finalists' stories from 2019 and 2020. The contest was created with a few goals in mind. First, we wanted to change the culture of fear around birth to one of solidarity, strength, and resilience. Second, we wanted to give voice to a diverse range of birthers, including those whose voices are often left out or underrepresented. Finally, we wanted to create awareness about doula support and its valuable place in perinatal care. To close out each year's birth story contest, we also held a Birth Sharing Circle—the first one in person, 2020's circle held virtually due to COVID-19. These circles united the jury and the finalists who shared their birth stories. We were blown away by the profound experience and solidarity those circles created among birthers through the power of compassionate listening, even when held online. The Birth Sharing Circle replays are available at https://www.doulasupport.org/book-page.

We are so happy to share a bouquet of birth stories in this book, including birth under varying circumstances and settings, with unexpected obstacles, and with different healthcare providers. Each story has its own voice, though they all centre on the voice of the birther. Each story shows vulnerability, strength, and love. A common thread in these stories is not only the birth of a new human being (even if preceded by loss in some cases), but also of parents, and the beginning of a love story. Like love stories, no two births are the same.

All of the birth stories we received during our Birth Story Writing Contests were stunning. In addition to highlighting the power and resilience of those who birth, many also shared heartwarming moments of birth workers who knew to provide just the right kind of support for the birthing person to feel safe, respected, and heard. Particularly in a world now familiar with realities of the COVID-19 pandemic, we see many birth workers on the frontlines who are overworked and underappreciated. We want to take a moment to express our gratitude to all of the nurses, midwives, obstetricians, and other healthcare providers who remain committed to facilitating positive and supported birthing experiences.

Through the reading of these birth stories, you will discover some Canadian published writers, emergent writers, and new writers who, taken together, have created a new language to describe labour and birth. All the non-medical jargon and well-crafted expressions create new imageries around labour and birth, which we hope will help shift us away from a fearful culture around birth to one of strength, respect, and resilience. Birth is so much more than a medical event—it is a critically transformative event in people's lives, and an event that every birther remembers forever. These stories bear witness to what a birth can be in Canada, and where more work is needed to ensure a positive birthing experience for all. After reading the birth stories, we provide additional information about holding Birth Sharing Circles of your own.

To situate the stories and provide essential ingredients for those preparing for birth and supporting those who birth, the second part of this book presents key evidence-based information about perinatal care. This includes information on healthcare provider and birth setting options, evidence on doula support, and understanding the unique challenges and realities that Indigenous, Black, and other people of colour face in birthing in Canada. We also include a section on the beginnings of breastfeeding, contributed by internationally renowned physician and breastfeeding expert Dr. Jack Newman and his colleague and award-winning author Teresa Pitman.

In addition to Newman and Pitman's valuable contribution, we are grateful to other key experts in Canadian perinatal care who contributed to our book. The foreword is written Dr. Michael Klein, a well-known and respected family physician, professor, and author of *The Dissident Doctor: My Life Catching Babies and Challenging the Status Quo*. Dr. Klein shares his experiences with and reflections on the life of Dr. Enkin, who pioneered the concept of evidence-based maternity care. Aboriginal midwife, Registered Midwife, and Professor Dr. Karen Lawford provides her valuable contributions shedding light on Indigenous communities and perinatal care, and Chandra Martini, an Alberta Registered Midwife and author of insightful research on Black pioneer midwives in Western Canada lends her wisdom by writing on how racial disparities and discrimination show up in the Canadian birthing context, and how we can all work together to create a more just and equal system that supports all people who birth. The other sections, on evidence on doula care, birth providers and settings, and perinatal care and human rights, are written by Doula Support Foundation doulas. To conclude the book, we had fun creating a "recipe for a satisfying birth," which can be summarized with one word: respect.

We want this book to be as beautiful as it is compelling and informative. Therefore, we peppered birth story-inspired artwork from local artists, as well as sprinkled quotes throughout the book to give some food for thought as well as a reading list of key books on pregnancy, labour, birth, and postpartum.

Although we have added to the voices of birthers, it is still their voices at the centre of this book. Our hope is that this book contributes to shaping a new culture surrounding birth; a culture that generates great respect for birthers and that celebrates their strength and resilience. We envision a culture that recognizes the needs for physical and emotional support before, during, and after this major life event, and one that expects nothing less than compassionate, patient-centred, and evidence-based care. As Kara Ananda writes in *Midwifery Today* (2011), "The power of a good birth story, regardless of how it is transmitted, is profound. Within our voices and stories is the power to change the culture of birth and bring healing."

We know that those stories will resonate a long time after you read them. We hope you savour them!

Josée Leduc, DSF'S Birth Story Writing Contest creator
Laura Pascoe, Doula Support Foundation co-founder

THE DOULA SUPPORT FOUNDATION: A SHORT STORY OF OUR BIRTH

by Laura Pascoe

When I became a doula, I knew I wanted to be a part of a community of doulas, a group with whom I could share with and learn from. I also hoped to join my voice with others who shared a common vision for supporting all those who birth to have positive and empowering birth experiences, regardless of income.

I was fortunate to find a small but inspired group of doulas in my then-local town of Kingston, Ontario who shared the same goals. We all spoke of a desire to build a collaborative and supportive doula community, to increase access to doula care, and to find a way to do so sustainably. So, we became a loosely defined collective. Over the next year (or thereabouts), we met regularly to share delicious potluck dinners and hash out our vision and longer-term plans. We quickly realized that there weren't many organizational models for how to get doula care to those who need it most without it coming out of the pockets of the doulas themselves. As doulas, we all agreed, we love what we do and have seen firsthand the value and impact of doula support. However, and just like nurses, personal support workers, massage therapists, and other professional providers of care and support, we recognized the importance of compensation for our efforts so we could focus our energy on our clients. In most places, doula support still isn't covered by health insurance, and we needed to find a model for care that got doulas paid without placing that burden on families already in financial duress.

So, towards the end of 2018, we founded the Doula Support Foundation, a registered not-for-profit serving Kingston, Ontario and the surrounding areas. The Doula Support Foundation (DSF) makes sustainable doula services available and accessible to all those who want them but could not otherwise afford them. Our long-term vision is to positively transform the experience of birth and parenting in our communities.

We are a doula organization aligned with reproductive justice, a term coined by the Black women-led SisterSong Women of Color Reproductive Justice Collective to define what it means to realize full reproductive health and freedom beyond a narrow understanding of "choice." Reproductive justice means achieving "the human right to maintain personal bodily autonomy, have children, not have children, and parent the children we have in safe and sustainable communities" (SisterSong, 2022). In our work, this includes providing the following types of doula support:

- Birth doulas
- Postpartum doulas
- Bereavement doulas for cases of pregnancy and infant loss, including termination of pregnancy (our *Prism* program)

We also knew that some of the clients most in need of support would be facing additional challenges, including substance use, mental health challenges, interactions with child welfare and protection services, and/or racial discrimination, among others. To help prepare our doulas to best support these clients, we developed additional training requirements (beyond each doula's certifying doula training) and organized topic-specific meetings to explore and reflect on these issues further, including inviting guest speakers with lived experiences and expertise they were willing to share.

Since we began, DSF Doulas have provided birth, postpartum, and loss support to close to 100 women and others who birth – and we're just getting started. As a non-profit organization, the financial support of our donors is paramount to our success in delivering doula support to those who need it most. You can donate at Doula Support Foundation | Donate. https://www.doulasupport.org/donate

We have also birthed other creative and impactful projects in line with our goals, namely the Birth Story Writing Contest, created and led largely by my co-editor and dear friend Josée Leduc. DSF remains a humble, primarily grassroots-funded organization that is run by dedicated volunteers. We have learned a lot along the way and know we have much more to learn. I am in awe of the incredible, resilient, thoughtful, brilliant, and compassionate doulas and other people who have been a part of DSF and continue to make our dream a reality. A huge thank you to all those who have contributed, whether past, present, or future, to the Doula Support Foundation and other organizations like it.

Laura Pascoe
Co-founder and former Chairperson of the Doula Support Foundation

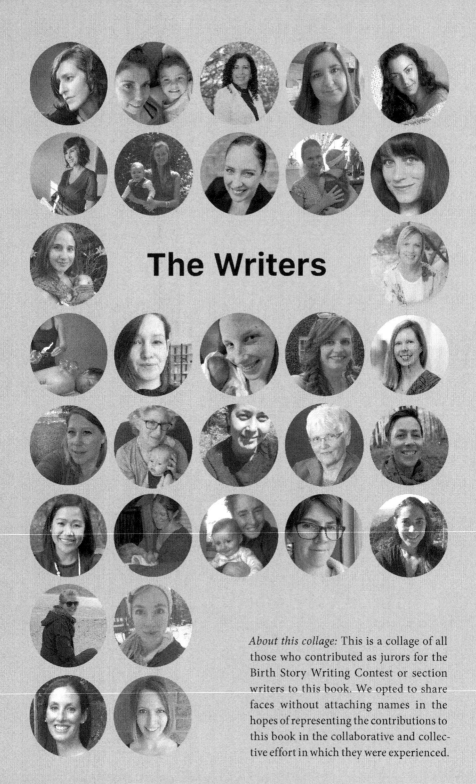

The Writers

About this collage: This is a collage of all those who contributed as jurors for the Birth Story Writing Contest or section writers to this book. We opted to share faces without attaching names in the hopes of representing the contributions to this book in the collaborative and collective effort in which they were experienced.

BIRTH STORIES

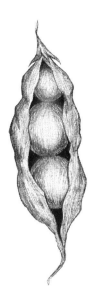

Labor and birth rate among the most intense of all normal human experiences, because they are so demanding- physically, emotionally and mentally. This is true not only for the person in labor, but also for those who love and care for that person. Labor is unpredictable, empowering and fulfilling- and it comes with a great prize at the end!

—Penny Simkin, *The Birth Partner*

Birth of the Tiger

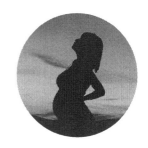

by **Ashley Lightfoot**
British Columbia
First-Place 2020

I look over the records.
That bottom section for Comments "if not normal"
Within, in midwife's script,
"Unattended home birth."

Diary Entry:

Thought I was in labour on Saturday, then again on Monday night.
Gotta just go with it.
Woke up at 4 a.m. and didn't feel the kick-kick-punch.
Got worried; couldn't sleep.
Ate till I felt movement, slow and lazy.
Not its usual self – losing space? Conserving energy?
Thirty-nine weeks tomorrow; moon waning.
Tiger, will you be a true new moon baby?
We'll go with your flow.

My second full-term babe.

This time around, we opted for early testing, and declined ultrasounds. The tiger evenswam away from the doppler at our first check-up, so we decided to use the fetoscope for the rest of the pregnancy. Blessed and thankful to be able to combine science and wisdom, and to be able to decide what works for our family. No paparazzi in the world of mom and babe. Just our language, our dreams, our hearts, all connected. I felt a bit silly, actually – a bit disappointed with myself to find I had more anxiety with this pregnancy despite feeling so well-informed. Then I was reminded, while flipping through a dog-eared copy of *Birthing from Within,* that worry is part of the work of pregnancy. This web of unknowns – shadow side of life, flip side of death. Magic.

I was ready. My first birth was long, at home, in water. Babe was looking upwards, head cocked to one side – asynclitic, brow-presentation. I felt invincible afterwards. The sensations had been so intense, the duration so exhausting. I had caressed the face of the creator. I was waiting for that again, for the hormones of the birth process to send me back to the space of Labourland. I knew that second labours were generally faster, but I didn't want to rely on it. My strategy was to mentally prepare for it to be more gruelling than the first. If it was easier, good. Gravy.

40 weeks, plus.

I went to a friend's farm with my kiddo.

In my pelvis, a tickle, like a balloon blowing up halfway and deflating.

Something.

I thought back to another friend's second babe and how her Braxton-Hicks went on for a week. We kept petting the horses, hardly convinced at all.

Later that afternoon, I told the husband I felt a bit unusual, but he should take our kid to swimming lessons.

"I've been asked to meet up for a beer…" he texted after the lesson.

"Sure, why not?"

Some spotting. A little mucus plug? A little cramping.

Then, I started working on my massive sewing pile.

Years-worth of sewing. Wait, what am I doing?

This is enough of a red flag that I text Jessica, my doula and mentor.

Legs a little numb.

It's about 4 p.m.

Bright red blood.

Interesting.

Sewing continues, and for some reason, I throw on *Scheherazade* as my background music.

The family returns and the husband makes dinner happen.

I'm not contributing to the household.

It's 7 p.m.,

Contracting.

But eating. I can't be *that* far along if I'm eating.

The world seems pretty normal.

Not going inward at all.

I request a doula visit. It's 8 p.m. and our kiddo is going to bed.

We talk till 8:30 p.m. I'm talking through contractions.

The mood is light.

"Would you like me to set up the birth pool?" Jessica asks.

"Well," I ponder, "the husband will want something to do, and I don't want to be a watched pot.

We'll call you. I'm going to have a shower."

Jess leaves, and while the husband is putting our eldest to bed, I text him an outline of tasks, with perfect spelling and grammar. So, *of course*, I'm nowhere near birthing.

I go to the bathroom not only to try to have a shower, but in the hopes of making some bowel room too. I mean, that's what you do, right? You poop and puke, and eventually, a baby comes out. Or, at least, that's what happened last time. I turn the shower on, but can't make it in. I'm floored by pain, gripping the side of the bathtub.

Then an excruciating stab on my left side puts me on all fours.

I still don't get it. I'm far too conscious.

Back from bedtime duties, the husband walks in, surveys, and wonders if I should get in the tub.

"I don't think I'll be able to get out again. I need to get to the bed, and where's my water bottle?"

I get into bed, water bottle in hand, and quickly realize that it's hard for me to put the cap back on.

"Text Jess; I'm gonna need someone to feed me water through a straw soon." (Finally, a sign that makes me realize I'm in a later stage of labour).

To ease my discomfort, I move to side-lying on my right side. I instruct the husband to inflate the birth pool, and soon after he leaves the room, the heavy-loud HUMMMMMMM of the electric air inflator whirrs up; it's the perfect muffle to the sudden mega-push that breaks my waters and moves the tiger's head right down with immense pressure (oh, and also voids my bowels quite prodigiously, at that). During that push, I had screamed the most primitive, murderous scream. As if the ambient air pump noise had helped get it all out of me. So primal, delicious, and kind of hilarious. Noticing the open window, I muse about what the neighbours can hear, and whether police services have been dispatched. Also, in that moment, I wonder, why am I still so freakin' with it? Where's my cosmic trip to search for life's ultimate truths?

The husband walks in, and basically sees that I have shit myself.

Understandably, this is his major concern.

So, he grabs a towel and starts cleaning up, bless.

What he's not yet aware of is that birth is here, furiously—I'm having some extreme hormone downloading, adrenaline spikes, and what feels like hours rolled into minutes.

Thinking and feeling is all I've got now, with brainwaves so slowed that words are not easy for me. I feel vortexed inward, sucked down to the underworld to emerge yet again as Mother.

All I can really say is, "Baby… baby."

He thinks *that's funny – she doesn't usually call me baby.*

Then he takes a closer look and shouts, "Is that *hair?*"

Not having signed up for this, he says, "I'm paging the midwives."

I'm too caught up to communicate my feelings, which, at the time are:

No, don't leave! I could kinda use you right now.

Another huge push takes me over.

There's a lot of pressure and I think *this is it!* So, I put my hand to my perineum, and *pop!*

Baby's head is out. Husband's yelling into the phone, "We have a head. We have a baby!"

It's been only 45 minutes from when I sent Jess packing.

He hangs up and comes over, surveying his second born's head sticking out of me.

"It's blue," he says.

"That's okay," I say.

"I think it's trying to say something! I think you need to push the rest of it out."

"Has it turned?" I ask.

"What?"

Having not really expected an unassisted birth, I had not briefed him in the mechanics of birth, which includes the very adept fetus rotating to most efficiently birth its shoulders.

I rephrase: "Has its head rotated yet?"

"What? I think you need to push it out."

Although I'm quite sure everything is actually going fine, I close my eyes and turn inward to search for another contraction, which I quickly found. It was like it met me on the astral plane, saying, "Oh, hello! I was almost there, but thanks for the company."

With that push, baby's torso comes out. Hips still in. It performs one more twist and my body pushes the rest out. Ta-da!

The husband puts the tiger on my chest. I gently rub, connect, and let the baby do what it needs to do. Some sputtering, and all is well. It knows my heart, my breast; it's home again. Cord pulsing, helping it switch over to this whole terrestrial breathing thing.

These next few minutes are a beautiful blur.

Jess shows up and the husband steps out for some air. Midwives soon after. I wish I could remember these moments better, hanging out with this new life. All I know was that 40 post-birth minutes feel like a flash. I'm asked if I need anything. I feel it's time for Dad to have some newborn skin-to-skin time. He gets in bed beside me. After all, that umbilical cord is attached to a baby, and that baby is still attached to a placenta, and that placenta has yet to be birthed. So, we have to be pretty close. Also, I would like that glass of red wine I've been wanting for months. I feel like a Viking Queen demanding my mead, and drink in that fashion.

The love hormones have effectively hotboxed the bedroom, and the victory drink has been tasted. Next comes talk that I should probably put some effort into birthing the placenta. So, I try to push. It feels huge, daunting. Harder than the birth.

Then, the husband pipes up. "Well, she birthed efficiently enough with you *not* here, so how about you all leave again?" As soon as the room clears, it slides out effortlessly. I'm so grateful for the husband stepping in to make sure I was given the space I needed. The perfect intimate advocate.

Placenta detached, it's time for a reset. I'm all for maintaining the hormonal aspects of birth, but this bed I've been on is covered in blood, amniotic fluid, and feces. And to a lesser extent, so am I. I go to the bathroom for a shower. I shake *so* hard. That was a tremendous fetal ejection. Still, I am buzzing with strength, unharmed, all parts intact and aware.

Soon after, Tiger gets weighed.

"Ten pounds, three ounces" the midwife exclaims.

Our cat sits proudly between the baby and placenta, and we prep the area for the umbilical cord burning but not before snapping a photo of the true knot in the cord, protected from tightening by Wharton's Jelly, and brilliant design. It's about 1 a.m. before the birth high wears off enough to consider sleep. Our birth keepers have refreshed the bed. Now, to sleep the gorgeous sleep of Mama and babe. Teaching new life how to breathe, feed, and the warmth of human touch – all of new life's necessities.

Over the next few days, life will return to its series of mundane tasks, with the 24/7 task of infant care piled on top. But not without some transcendent moments of bliss. My first postpartum was, like many, awash with this extraordinary newness, as well as a somewhat terrifying, hyper-alert sense of responsibility. This time around, I found moments where I felt truly bathed in the elementary particles of bonding. The husband was home keeping house, the neighbours brought food and didn't linger, a friend even provided acupuncture to ease my post-labour pains. With all of that beautiful support, I was left to do this important work, relaxed enough to receive the pure spiritual simplicity of love between baby and birther.

The husband and I still sit back sometimes and start debriefing on that night. We pull the memory out as one would an after-dinner treat from the freezer.

"You manifested that," he says.

I purr with appreciation for our union and what it has created.

So, there you have it – the birth of the tiger.

It wasn't the story we thought we'd be telling.

In birth, as in life, is it ever?

2021 Update: *This story is dedicated to the memory of Jessica Austin, passionate birth worker, advocate, teacher, fiercely loving mother, and wife whose old soul guided so many during her brief and powerful time, earthside.*

About Ashley

When not running around with her two young kidlets, Ashley is attending births as a doula, writing custom lullabies for new babies, out on a paddleboard, or flying planes at the local airport. She is a member of the BC Doula Services Association and serves on the board of the Tantalus Wellspring Society, a charity that assists those experiencing barriers in accessing mental wellness therapies. She can be reached at www.moonbeamdoula.ca.

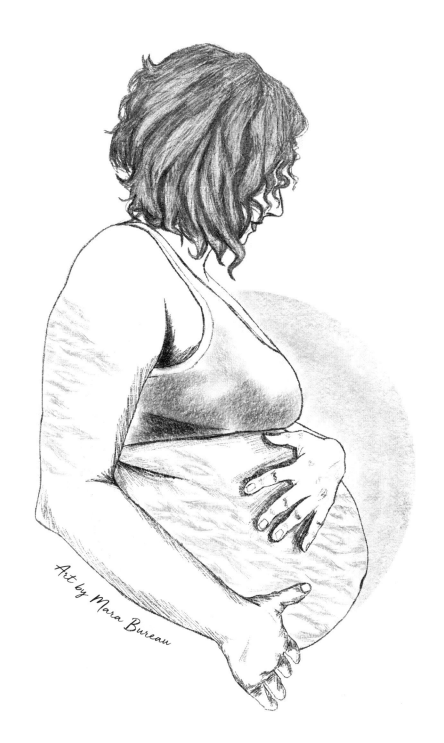

A Blazing Birth

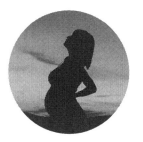

by Mandee MacDonald
Napanee, Ontario
First Place 2019

"You don't want to have this baby in the car," my doctor joked at my prenatal appointment, referring to the speed at which my first was delivered and the fact that second births can be even faster.

Imagine that, having a baby in the car…

Now *that* could be traumatizing.

We were ecstatic about expecting our second. I loved him already. Daddy would get a son and my daughter would become a big sister.

The pregnancy was progressing as expected. With my first pregnancy, I was a huge worrywart, fretting about what I ate and how I moved and the positions in which I slept. But with my second, I was much more relaxed.

Despite my firstborn being nine days late, I found myself in early labour in my 38th week with my little boy. After having contractions increase and then taper off for a couple of days, I made an appointment with my doctor for that evening. Our 20-month-old was at Grandma's, which worked out well when I found out at my appointment that I was over 2 cm dilated.

We got some pizza and movies and were enjoying our time together while we waited for the contractions to progress. It was exciting, imagining that it could be the night we'd meet our newest addition. Jordan, my husband, did some massage on my back to the point that I couldn't even time the contractions anymore. His technique worked so well that I couldn't feel when they started and when they ended. We were chill and relaxed that evening, optimistic about meeting our son, and having no idea what was about to happen.

Throughout the evening, we discussed whether we should head to the hospital, but we kept waiting until the contractions intensified. Finally, we decided that we would lie down for 30 minutes, timing the contractions to know whether they were increasing or find out if they were slowing down. We lay down, Jordan started reading a book, and I waited.

Suddenly, a contraction enveloped me in pain, holding me tightly for many seconds. It felt different, more intense, and it held me tighter as I waited for it to end.

"Okay, we're going!" my husband said, as I recovered from the contraction, and I didn't argue with him. I was ready to go.

It was official. We were heading to the hospital! The excitement of the occasion, the nerves of the unknown, and the anticipation of meeting our baby boy was setting in.

For about 10 minutes, Jordan swiftly attended to the details (informing his mom, getting the bags, moving the cars), but suddenly, unexpectedly, the urgency intensified. Instead of being patient, calm, and relaxed, a feeling of panic grew that told me, *we need to go now.* The excitement was replaced by fear – fear of not making it in time; being alone when having a baby; not knowing what to do; facing the pain myself. Pleading for him to hurry, I stepped out into the dark winter night, and we rushed off in the car.

The contractions were increasing relentlessly without much break in between. I quickly dialled my doula and then gripped the car as we sped off into the night. At first, my doula calmly explained that she could head out to meet us at the hospital.

Then I told her, "I feel like I'm peeing myself."

She heard my pain in my voice and she quickly deduced that Jordan needed to pull over. Out of fear, we kept driving. What if we didn't make it in time? What if something happened?

At that moment, I started feeling a sensation, a strong urge similar to needing to use the washroom, and I clamped it back. The pressure continued, with me resisting and squeezing back, but each time, it got stronger. My doula told me to call 911.

In that moment of confusion, the darkness and coldness of the night, Jordan speeding down the road, my doula insisting over the phone that we pull over, my holding on and trying to resist the feeling that something was coming out, the intensity of the fear… we knew we were about to birth our miracle.

I tried to explain the situation to the emergency services. I gave a general location and explained that I was about to give birth, but then I quickly hung up so that I could call my doula back.

But the pressure came on again, and this time, something different happened. I did not hold it in, I did not keep it back, I did not make it stop. Then, it happened. Amid the fear, the uncertainty, the reluctance, there was a feeling of release. The sensation overwhelmed my efforts to squeeze it back, and in that surreal moment, I felt it all come out.

"Jordan, he's out!" I exclaimed as we whizzed past Richardson Stadium. A soft crying could be heard from my pants.

Jordan, hands on the steering wheel, darted his eyes in my direction and witnessed his slimy little son in his wife's stretchy black leggings. He turned the car around and pulled into Richardson Stadium.

My doula told us to wrap him in Jordan's jacket to keep him warm, but I hesitated. I was so scared that he was not okay. In that moment, with the rush of adrenaline, I could not bring myself to physically reach down and touch him. The fear crippled me.

Jordan came to my side of the car and picked him up, unwrapping the umbilical cord that was wrapped loosely around his neck. It was that moment when my maternal instincts kicked in and I told Jordan to give him to me so we could do skin-on-skin. My doula instructed us not to cut the cord, to keep him warm, and to rub him until he cried.

The ambulance arrived rather quickly and whisked the baby and me off to the hospital. Jordan followed behind, repeating, "No, he's really here already!" over the phone to my mom's disbelief. Upon arrival, we were greeted by numerous hospital staff, and we felt like little celebrities.

So, there we were, a family of four before we even arrived at the hospital. The doctors and nurses reaffirmed that Blaze and I were fine.

Ironically, the name "Blaze" had been chosen prior to his birth, but the birth, of course, fit perfectly with our choice.

That delicate instance when Blaze arrived—an experience only the three of us shared, unexpectedly—bonded us as a couple and as a family in a way that we never would have expected. That night was over four years ago now. This event changed our lives. The details that characterized those moments forever remain etched on our hearts.

All of my kids came into this world in unique but amazing ways. The first baby came while I laughed at the way everyone around me was smiling with each push and my lack of pain due to the epidural; the second came on the way to the hospital; the third one came before the doctor had time to put her second glove on; and the final one fell into the nurse's hands as I was standing up. Each story has shaped us as a family, taught us about parenthood, forced us to trust, and prepared us for raising them in a unique way. It signified their very first moments in the world and it was perfect.

I came to the profound realization that my body was created and designed to do something spectacular. On that February night, it brought new life into the world without any prodding, pushing, or monitoring, and despite a whole lot of resistance on my end.

I would not advocate for doing that again. In fact, I made a point to be at the hospital on time with my last baby, and I was. But I am so thankful to God that there were not any complications that required immediate medical attention and that I was given such a gift in the unexpected. It wasn't traumatizing at all – it was miraculous.

In the dark of that winter night, we became a family of four – swiftly, uniquely, but perfectly.

Your birth story, whether unexpected or as planned, equips you for all the uncertain moments in parenting. The times you question yourself; the days you wonder what the right choice is; the instances when things do not go as planned.

We let those parenting moments shape us so that one day, when we look back on them, we are proud of the things we accomplished and never knew we could.

Quite honestly, being able to look back and see the feat that you accomplished, the journey your body completed, and the growth that came from it, well, that is the most amazing birth story anyone could ask for.

For us, to this day, it makes driving past Richardson Stadium just a little more interesting.

So, from now on, if anyone around us admits their fear of having a baby in a car or not making it to the hospital, Jordan and I can look at each other, smiling, sharing an intimate twinkle in our eye that only we can understand.

"You never know," I would say, shrugging my shoulders. "It happens."

About Mandee

Mandee MacDonald lives in Napanee, Ontario. She is a Queen's University and Southeastern University alumni. She is also a hairstylist and a teacher, but at the moment, she is a stay-at-home mom to four little ones. So, these days, she changes diapers, makes peanut butter sandwiches, and watches *Paw Patrol*. The days aren't always glamorous, but she counts being a mom as one of her greatest accomplishments.

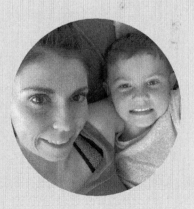

Cutting Ties and Letting Go

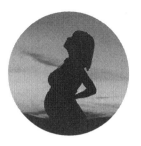

by Lori Sebastianutti
Stoney Creek, Ontario
Second-Place 2020

There were two men in the room when I got pregnant: one holding my hand and the other at the base of my stirrup-bound feet. A woman pressed a cold ultrasound wand on my lower abdomen and another man passed a catheter through a small window from an adjoining room. It wasn't the most romantic setting, but no less miraculous.

I got pregnant with my first child after seven and a half years of trying and multiple in-vitro fertilization (IVF) procedures. The reproductive endocrinologist (RE) who helped us achieve this feat was not the first one we saw, but we wanted him to be the last, so we stuck through four years and five IVF transfers before we saw those coveted two pink lines.

After our 12-week ultrasound, we got his clearance to have our care transferred to an OB/GYN.

"Can we stay with you?" I asked.

I knew that, in addition to performing fertility procedures, he was also practicing obstetrics. It had been painful seeing pregnant women exit examination rooms while I left with a flat belly and hundreds of dollars worth of fertility drugs.

"Sure," he said. "But your baby will be born at Joe Brant Hospital."

I tried to not let it bother me that my child would be the first in a family of Italian immigrants who settled in Hamilton, Ontario to have "Burlington" listed as his place of birth on his birth certificate. I didn't want to start over with someone new, not after we had come so far. Would a frightened child let go of their parent's hand in a crowded room?

The pregnancy would be marked by two distinct features: hyperemesis gravidarum and anxiety. I refused to take medication for either and I simply pushed through. Round-the-clock nausea and vomiting relented at 20 weeks, but the anxiety persisted until the day I gave birth and beyond. At every turn during those 40 weeks and 5 days, I thought something would go wrong. Was I really going to be a mother after almost eight years? Was this just a cruel joke? I was convinced that one day, I would wake up and realize that it had all been a dream. I would be back on the other side of the window, face pressed up against the glass, watching all the mothers rock, nurse, and care for their precious babies.

But it was real, and I wanted to be as prepared as I could. My husband and I took two birthing classes: one offered by the hospital and the other by a doula that had been my counsellor during the last two years of my infertility journey. A specialist in hypnosis, she tried to help me uncover any barriers that were preventing my body from achieving pregnancy. The medical diagnosis of "unexplained infertility" had done nothing to provide answers, so for two years, we worked through affirmations and visualizations, and she listened to me cry when yet another friend or a family member became pregnant with ease. Now that I was on the other side, I wanted to work with her during her hypnobirthing classes to support the mind-body connection during the birthing process.

While I did my best to absorb the myriad of information presented in both classes, the only true goal that I had for the birth of my first child was to deliver him vaginally. Infertility had robbed me of so much: the chance to follow a projected timeline for my life, the opportunity to fit in with my peer group, and most significantly, the ability to achieve a spontaneous conception.

With a vaginal delivery, I hoped to witness the power of my body in a way that women had been experiencing for millennia. I was, however, open to the idea of a C-section if it was deemed medically necessary. The health and safety of my child would veto any feelings about the way I hoped he would come into the world. I had full faith in a doctor who had given us the chance to be in this position in the first place. How could a miracle worker steer me wrong?

At 40 weeks, my doctor decided to schedule an induction. In five days, he would be on call, and he knew how much I wanted him to be the doctor to deliver my child. He had been there when my son went in, and my husband and I wanted him to be there when he came out.

The day before the induction, he had me come to the hospital to have progesterone gel applied to encourage dilation. The next morning, my cervix was measured at 1 cm, and I had antibiotics administered through an IV, as I had tested positive for Strep B. After a sufficient amount of time, my doctor broke my water, and a nurse started the Pitocin drip while my husband, my mother, and I waited for contractions to begin.

Begin, they did. From the outset, they came fast and furious, not slow and controlled as I had learned in my birthing classes. Almost immediately, I felt as though my insides were being squeezed so tight that I thought I might explode and fall into pieces on the hospital floor like a popped balloon.

Despite my constant pleas for an epidural, I was told that the anesthetist was in a complicated surgery and since he was the only one on call, I would have to wait. For the next five hours, I cried, screamed, and threw up until he finally walked through the door.

"I bet you're happy to see me," he said. The tears rolling down my cheeks were my answer.

After two attempts to get the medication started, I lay in bed, watching my contractions on a screen while feeling nothing but comfort. I took a short nap and when I woke to intense pressure on my bowels, I notified the nurse. She told me that she would call the doctor, as this indicated to her that it was time to push.

I began pushing with the nurse holding one leg and my husband holding the other. When the doctor made his way into the room all suited up, he told me I may need forceps or vacuum extraction to help my son descend. Determined to avoid both of those scenarios, I pushed with all the might I could muster.

After an hour, my doctor told me I was going to need an episiotomy. I vaguely remembered the word from the birthing classes. I knew it meant my vagina would have to be cut to help my son's head escape. It didn't sound pleasant, but I trusted my doctor wholeheartedly.

"Okay," I said between pushes.

After numbing the area with local anesthesia, he used a pair of surgical scissors to make a small incision to my perineum and posterior vaginal wall. My husband said he remembers a large squirt of blood escape like water from a burst pipe. With the next push, my son was out, and eight years of struggle and heartache unleashed into a torrent of tears. As they were examining my son, and after I had been stitched up, I grasped my doctor's hand and thanked him between sobs.

There is one word that characterized the days and weeks after the delivery of my first child: pain. I couldn't sit, walk, or move in any way without feeling a pulsating ache in the most intimate part of my body. Nurses were changing shifts every 12 hours telling me to sit up and walk around. My small room was constantly filling and emptying of well-meaning family members and friends.

Emotional pain soon followed, as I found breastfeeding next to impossible. In the first 24 hours, my son needed little nourishment, but as his appetite grew, my inability to relax and ignore the pain prevented any real progress. I asked a nurse for stronger medication than the extra strength ibuprofen and acetaminophen I was interchanging every four hours, but she told me it was "doctor's orders." Anything stronger would be incompatible with breastfeeding. My husband fed him his first bottle of formula as I looked on from the bed trying to ignore the large rock in my chest.

During one of my physical exams, a nurse told me my incision was healing beautifully.

"But I'm in so much pain," I said.

She nodded. "It's a small incision, but he cut through four layers of tissue. That's why you feel it so much."

After three days of regular Sitz baths and squirt bottle cleanings, we left the hospital with a thriving newborn. What followed was intense guilt and depression over the inability to push through the pain of my episiotomy and breastfeed my son.

One night, while my parents were visiting, I quietly escaped to the nursery and tried to put him to the breast. He struggled to latch and began to wail. My mother entered the room with a small bottle of formula and passed it to me. As tears streamed down my cheeks, she asked what was wrong.

"I'm a failure," I said. "I couldn't feed him with my body."

"Look at him," she urged.

I looked down at my hard-fought baby with his round face, wide eyes, and pink cheeks.

"How can anyone who made him be a failure?" she said.

In psychology, the term *transference* refers to the redirection of a patient's feelings for a significant person to the therapist or doctor. When the feelings are overly positive, it is called "God Syndrome." This occurs when the doctor is overvalued and becomes a type of god in the eyes of the patient.

I didn't think of my RE as a god, but in my mind, he was a miracle worker. This allowed me to put all my trust in him. The medical community came through when I needed it the most. How could it possibly lead me astray?

The emotional wound left by my episiotomy took much longer to heal than the physical one. Eventually, I shifted my thinking, which allowed me to put more faith in myself than any medical professional. Now it was my turn to do the cutting.

When I turned 39, my husband and I were ready to try for baby number two. Knowing that time was not on our side, we switched doctors. I began treatments in a clinic with higher-than-average success rates for women over 37 who wanted to use their own eggs.

To our delight, I became pregnant after four months. This time, when my RE asked me if I had any preference for my obstetrical care, I was prepared. I asked to be referred to a female team of obstetricians in Hamilton who rarely performed episiotomies, except in particular cases.

With my second son, I only pushed for 20 minutes and had two surface tears that I barely noticed. His birth prompted further reflection that, even though I may not have had an episiotomy, if I had given birth at another hospital with a different doctor, it was okay. I chose to be gentle with myself, knowing that vulnerability was a logical state for me to be in after an almost eight-year struggle to become pregnant.

I'm glad I got a second chance at giving birth. My first time didn't turn out quite as I hoped it would, but it put in motion the long process of learning to have faith in an imperfect body. It's still a work in progress, but I realize that I can be grateful to others and self-trusting at the same time. Today, I choose to see the divine in a mind that can decide for itself and a body that can work miracles.

About Lori

Lori Sebastianutti is a writer of creative nonfiction. Her personal essays explore feminism, fertility, and faith. Her work has been published in *The New Quarterly*, *The Humber Literary Review*, and *The Hamilton Review of Books*, among others. You can read more of her work at https://lorisebastianutti.com and follow her on Instagram @sebastianlwrites.

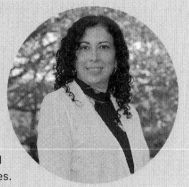

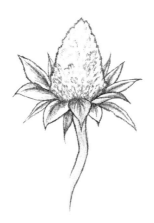

Grief is a force of energy that cannot be controlled or predicted. It comes and goes on its own schedule. Grief does not obey your plans, or your wishes. Grief will do whatever it wants to you, whenever it wants to. In that regard, Grief has a lot in common with Love.

　—**Elizabeth Gilbert,** TED Interviews podcast
https://www.themarginalian.org/2018/10/17/elizabeth-gilbert-ted-podcast-love-loss/

A Healing Birth

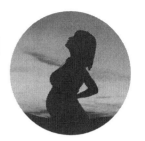

by Karen Price
Kingston, Ontario
Second-Place 2019

This is the story of how I came to have one of the most special boys in the world. The story begins back in April of 2008. I was 22 weeks pregnant at the time. On April 18th, while I was at work, I noticed that I had started bleeding. I contacted my husband and he left work immediately to pick me up. He rushed me to the hospital. where we were whisked up to the maternity floor. Right away, I was hooked up to monitors, an IV, and an ultrasound was ordered.

It didn't take long before they took us to have the ultrasound. This is when we got the news that we were having a boy. After a few minutes, the technician went to get the doctor, who came right in to tell us that they found a 14 cm blood clot in with the baby. They could not find any reason for the blood clot to be there but guessed it might have been a partial placental abruption. It was unusual and nothing specific happened to cause this. They informed us that there was nothing to be done, labour had begun, and they couldn't stop it.

They moved us to a private birthing room and prepared us to give birth to a baby boy we couldn't keep. At 22 weeks, he was too small; he would not be considered viable. The pediatrician told us that if he survived the labour, we could hold him until he passed away. I was given an epidural for the pain and morphine to sedate me, and on April 19th at 1:33 a.m., I gave birth to my baby boy, Benjamin. He was 1 lb, 1 oz, and the most perfect little baby. He, unfortunately, did not survive the birth, but we were able to hold him and say our goodbyes. There is no real way to properly express the devastation and immense sorrow we felt during this time. Robb was my rock; he kept me sane. We will forever be grateful for our nurse, Chris, during this labour. She provided a lot of comfort to Robb and me, as she had been through a similar situation herself and went on to have three healthy pregnancies and deliveries.

The hospital moved us to a private room while I recovered. Robb and I were visited by a social worker. She spent some time with us talking about what had happened and making sure we were on the path to healing. I remember her saying that she knew we would be okay just by watching us. She could see that there was no blame or hurt towards each other, which often happens in these situations. Without all the support, I don't know how I would have coped.

Time passes, the pain eases, but it never goes away completely. We discovered that we were pregnant again. We were thrilled, but terrified. I made an appointment with my OB right away and met with his resident. She took a keen interest in us due to my history and recommended that we consult Dr. John Kingdom, a renowned placental specialist.

Due to our loss, we were hesitant to share the news and decided to wait until after we had our appointment with Dr. Kingdom that was scheduled for when I was 20 weeks along.

When the time finally came, we started the process of numerous ultrasounds and tests. When completed, he sat us down in his office to tell us that I had Vasa Previa. Vasa Previa is a rare condition where the fetal umbilical vessels are lying along the cervix and affects about 1 in 2000 pregnancies. If it is undetected, just under half will survive. He was pleased that we were able to discover it early because that increases the survival rate to 97%.

I would have to have a C-section to deliver—there was no way around that—and I would have to give birth at 36 or 37 weeks to ensure I didn't go into labour. His confidence in his ability to take us through this pregnancy and give us a baby at the end was reassuring, but we were terrified. Dr. Kingdom put me on modified bed rest. I couldn't work and basically, all I could do was go from my bed to the couch.

After what had happened with Benjamin, we were too scared to get anyone else excited, and really didn't want to have to explain what happened if anything went wrong. This news made it even more difficult to tell anyone. We told close family members what was happening, but mostly kept the news to ourselves until we were 24 weeks along.

The rest of the pregnancy passed uneventfully with long periods of boredom and several doctor appointments. During all of these visits, we found out that we were expecting another boy. We decided to name him Dexter Earl.

Our C-section was scheduled for April 1st, 2009. The night before, we stayed in a hotel in downtown Toronto so that we could make it to Mt. Sinai Hospital without having to deal with the traffic. We arrived at the hospital the morning of April 1st and we were quickly prepped and taken to the OR. Mt. Sinai is a teaching hospital and Dr. Kingdom had asked if we would allow some of his residents to observe the C-section. I was more than happy to let people learn from my experience so that they could save lives. In addition to Dr. Kingdom and his five residents in the operating room were an anesthesiologist, a NICU nurse with an incubator (just in case), and a nurse that just stood with me to make sure I was feeling okay for the duration of the procedure.

Dr. Kingdom started the procedure and asked if we had chosen a name. We told him the name we had chosen, and in less than five minutes, he delivered Dexter. When he held him up, everyone in the room cheered and said, "Hello, Dexter!" That is when he let out a giant wail and I felt the biggest sigh of relief in 36 weeks.

Dr. Kingdom placed Dexter on the warming table and walked away, leaving him there. He then started teaching a lesson about placenta previa to his residents. He asked Robb if he had brought a camera because he would like a picture of my placenta saying, "It is the most perfect example of placenta previa" he had ever seen. Robb was unwilling to take the pictures himself, so he gave our camera to one of the nurses. He went over to the warming table and crouched down beside Dexter and started stroking his back and talking to him. The relief and joy had me crying as I watched him with our baby. Robb was the first one to hold him and brought him over to me so I could finally see him up close.

We spent the rest of the time in the OR laughing and crying while Robb held him. Once we were taken to recovery, I finally could hold him. Robb took that opportunity to call our families to let them know the newest member of our family was safely with us. During our time in the hospital, Dexter lived in my housecoat like a little kangaroo; he was happiest whenever he could be right against my skin. We spent three days in the hospital recovering. The doctors and nurses at Mt. Sinai were amazing. They were able to answer all of our questions and spent lots of time with us giving us all the help we needed.

Dexter Earl was 6 pounds, 15 ounces, and 20 inches long. We will forever miss the possibilities we could have had with Benjamin but are forever grateful for all the opportunities we have had with Dexter.

Maybe I should add that following Dexter, I had one miscarriage and one normal pregnancy. Regardless of being told that there was nothing wrong, Robb and I walked on eggshells for the entire pregnancy waiting for something to go wrong. Fortunately, my second son, Elliot Louis, was born healthy by a planned C-section on March 2nd, 2011.

Pregnancy has been a stressful time for me. I have always been envious of the people who seem to breeze through pregnancy and labour, never once having to think that it may not work out. But I can say with utmost certainty that my boys bring me so much joy every day and I anticipate many more years of joy and memories with them. I will always be grateful to the doctors and nurses that have helped us deliver our boys safely.

About Karen

Karen Price lives in Kingston, Ontario. She is new-ish to the Kingston area and works for the Limestone School Board. She has two sons, ages 11 and 8.

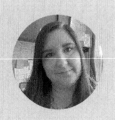

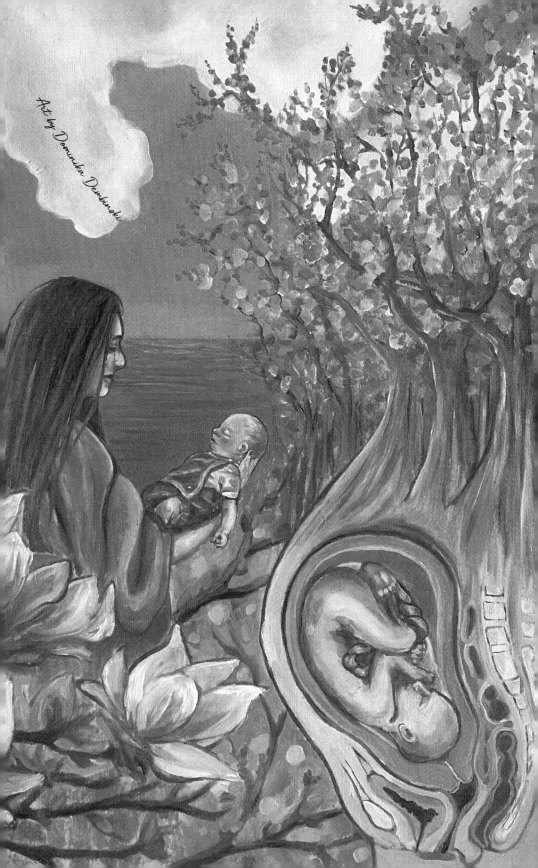

Luna Rising

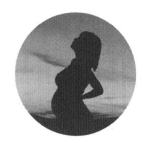

by Mercedes Papalia
York, Ontario
Third-Place 2020

It's 3 a.m. and I'm wrapped in a blanket, looking out the front window of our Toronto bungalow. My body mirrors the full pink moon revealing her magnificence through the gently swaying branches of the tree standing proudly on our lawn. This lunar phase carries the powerful energy of rebirth and inspires transformation and recognition that we are cyclic beings in conjunction with nature.

"Ah, of course," I whisper to the moon. "She was waiting for you. How poetic, my Luna."

Today marks two weeks past her expected date of arrival. The house is quiet. I peek into the bedroom to see my husband TJ comfortably cuddled up with our little dog, Toby. The floor squeaks as my swollen feet slowly move me into Luna's nursery. Her crib is covered in sheets freshly washed by my mom and adorned with a macramé banner handmade by one of our closest friends.

On the floor is a plastic blue bin filled to the brim with every suggested item on the checklist from my midwife. Eight towels, check; four receiving blankets, check; two bowls, check; a metal baking sheet, check. My diaper bag, however, is practically empty. This is a home birth. I've read Ina May's *Spiritual Midwifery*, and I am ready for initiation into the "badass women who've birthed their babies naturally" club. I hold this idea like a badge of honour I'll soon be wearing.

"This isn't that bad!" I tell TJ as he makes coffee with a subtle jitter in his hands.

Soon, my doula Asma arrives, wide-eyed, calm, and genuinely excited to be here. Asma shares the birth stories of her two children as I bounce on an oversized exercise ball. I exhale in revelation of the honour it is to have Asma here supporting me with real compassion and sisterhood.

I rest. I bathe. I bounce. I walk. I rest. I snack. I hug my husband. I rest. I kiss my husband. I bathe. I snack. I notice Asma through the crack of the nursery door sitting on my brand-new rocking chair pumping breast milk. *Wow,* I say to myself under my breath. I walk. I snack. I rest.

Over the next 24 hours, the pain increases steadily. I eventually surrender and wrap my body around a pile of pillows in agony. My newly arrived midwife Sarah sits at the foot of my bed. She explains that because my water hasn't broken, I can choose to have her break it or wait. She tells me it could take anywhere from a few hours to another day or two, and gently warns that if she breaks my water, the pain will increase rapidly. I laugh, because worse than this is simply not possible. I ask to see what she will put inside me to break my water. It looks like one of those things my grandparents use to put their shoes on.

"Okay, let's do it," I say.

Then like a transport truck in a highway collision, it happens. *This* must be the most pain a human can maybe survive. I get back on my hands and knees. My voice generates sounds that derive from deeper than the depth of my womanhood. They were no longer mine; they are that of an animal awoken within.

I look up toward my bedroom door between excruciating surges. My husband stands there, and he too seems to have transformed from a broad six-foot man to a 6-year-old boy. Terrified. Shaking. His ocean eyes puffy and red, his shirt soaked from tears; he watches me, desperately wanting to take my pain away.

"Babe," I say, as I grab his head and pull him toward me. "This is hard, and I'm scared too, but I'm okay. I know it doesn't look like it, but I'm okay. I'm going to give birth to our daughter."

A fire of gratitude ignites in my soul. He isn't pretending to hold it together. He's just here, terrified, trusting me, loving me.

Sarah comes in for another checkup, I assume because the sounds coming out of me have deepened once again. She's gentle and quiet, yet serious, like the CEO of my vagina hosting an important meeting. She tells me I'm 9 cm dilated, and that Lu's head seems to have dropped. This is it.

I call upon my courage to prepare my body for the next stage of labour and–

"Whoa." I pause.

The pain has disappeared. What? How? I lie to Asma; I tell her the surges are still terrible and exaggerate my moans to match what they were.

Sarah investigates. Then, I watch as she places her hand gently on mine.

"Mercedes, your cervix has closed, and you are 3 cm dilated," she says.

I don't want to believe her, but my body already knew. I pull my sweat-drenched spaghetti strap dress over my head and step into a lukewarm shower. As the water pours over my body, I feel physically, emotionally, and spiritually depleted. There's nothing left in me except the big ball of human that I am incapable of birthing.

I cry. I cry so hard that the stream of water coming from the faucet seems to merge with my tears.

After what feels like a lifetime, I catch my breath and pray, "Universe, God, whoever or whatever you are, please help me."

I crawl into bed and try to sleep for the first time in two days.

The clock says it's 1 p.m., but I don't know what day it is. My contractions are a few minutes apart and becoming more and more difficult to manage. For the first time, I'm really scared. My gut is speaking clearly to me; I know it's time to go to the hospital. I'm clinging to the hurtful backlash I felt from the outside world when I first decided to have a home birth.

My ego boldly argues, *if you go, you prove them right*. My soul whispers adamantly, *go to the hospital*.

I crawl into the back of our green Civic, Yolanda the Honda. TJ is not crying. He has a job to do and helping me is where TJ thrives. I feel his confidence as he gets behind the wheel. He safely swerves and speeds through the back roads, repeating, "You're doing great, babe!" Just like they do in the movies. I'm on my hands and knees, exploding with long deep cries of distress. I'm using swear words I didn't know were in my vocabulary. I can no longer recognize where one ends and the other begins. It's just one long, viscous feeling, beginning in my uterus and shooting through my entire body and beyond.

When we get to St. Joseph's Hospital, I climb onto the sterile bed and cry to my midwife, "It's too bright and I'm too tired." Then, I mutter through tears, "I think I need an epidural. I don't know if my body can handle it anymore. I'm sorry, I'm so sorry I can't do it."

For me, in this moment, asking for an epidural means failure. Sarah tells me I *am* doing it and that I'm incredibly strong and brave. I don't believe her.

I've been given a gas mask [nitrous oxide] and it is my new most favourite invention in the history of the world. I'm convinced that TJ and I are part of a secret society, and he can hear my thoughts as I tap my nose and raise my eyebrows repeatedly at him. I feel myself floating above my body. I can still feel the pain, but it feels like someone else's. This is better than sex.

Sarah's dark eyes pop up from between my legs.

"Mercedes!" she says, with a mildly excited tone. "I can see her head!"

I quickly pull off the mask and ask, "What colour is her hair?"

Through desperation and pain surpassing anything I could have ever imagined, I want to know the colour of my daughter's hair.

Sarah then says, "It's wet, so hard to tell, but there's lots of it," in a tone that accidentally embarrasses me for asking. "Are you ready to push?"

The epidural hasn't shown up. I feel everything as hands reach inside me to pull Luna down. Hands. Two hands and a baby all inside me. I'm pushing and they're pulling and it's happening. Then suddenly, a familiar nothing.

No Luna. Just a half dozen women (when did they multiply?) standing around, looking at my vagina. Some holding my legs, some writing things down, some just watching me. I look at the huge red and black digital clock in the corner of the room. I can't recall what the numbers were earlier, but I know time has passed.

A tiered cart filled with medical instruments pushed by a slender, serious-looking man rolls past me. I decide immediately that he is mean and terrible. I do not like that I need what he's preparing to stick into my spine. I sit with my legs dangling off the side of the hospital bed. My favourite intern midwife, Caitlin, senses my vulnerability and invites me to wrap my arms around her. With my head on her chest, she strokes my hair and gently explains what will happen next.

A green-eyed nurse with a tiny frame and frizzy red hair adjusts the needle taped to my skin.

"I can still feel everything. Can you make it so I feel less?" I plead quietly.

"Yes, I will try," she replies. Just like that, the pain has gone from 100 out of 10 to 40 out of 10. "The doctor is here," she says softly.

The what?! I think to myself. *I did not sign up for any doctor. I don't even want to be here, I* **hate**- and a vivacious dark-haired woman in scrubs interrupts my thought. She oozes confidence bridging on arrogance and I like it.

"Hello, love, I'm Dr. Maria. Let's meet this baby, shall we?"

Luna's heart rate is dropping and so is mine. Dr. Maria is between my knees, holding large metal forceps as midwives grasp my bent legs. TJ stands just behind them, and Asma beside him.

The visceral support I'm feeling from each human in this room is palpable. Somehow, this sensation expands, and I am held by every female in the entire history of existence who has given birth before this moment. This powerful force shifts me to laser-sharp focus. I push with every ounce of strength I have as Dr. Maria pulls until, finally, Luna.

The biggest little hands stretch toward me and our deep brown eyes lock for the first time.

"She looks like my dad!" I cry.

I feel each stitch carefully being sewn, as Dr. Maria casually says something about "next time." We make a 10-dollar bet that there will be no next time. Asma takes photos of Luna's first moments as I ask repeatedly for my mom and family. I'm told to wait, as my placenta has not made her debut yet. Seriously? What feels like a lifetime later, I push the complex organ out of my body that allowed my daughter to grow inside me. It's so big that it rips my stitches. At this point, nothing surprises me.

I request that my 6-year-old niece, Ellia, be allowed in the room first. Caitlin asks Ellia to help her check Luna's heartbeat and I'm happy that she feels special. I hold my mom's hand while Luna lays on me. It feels so natural that I'm certain we've been together for lifetimes.

"Happy Birthday, my love," I say quietly into her tiny ear.

It's been 65 hours since the subtle surge that woke me up. None of this is what I expected, planned for, or dreamed of. It is nothing like the stories I read, but it is mine. This is the beginning of the greatest adventure, the deepest love affair, and the most incredible journey of my life.

About Mercedes

Mercedes is a multi-disciplinary storyteller through art, design, and creative writing. Though her journey began as vocalist and actor, she continues to expand and diversify her practices. Mercedes currently resides on a tiny island on the West coast of Canada, where she can be found gardening, creating, and working as an Intuitive Mentor to artists across the country. She is a devoted mother, wife, and lover of fresh flowers and authentic Italian food, forever in the pursuit of her most beautiful life.

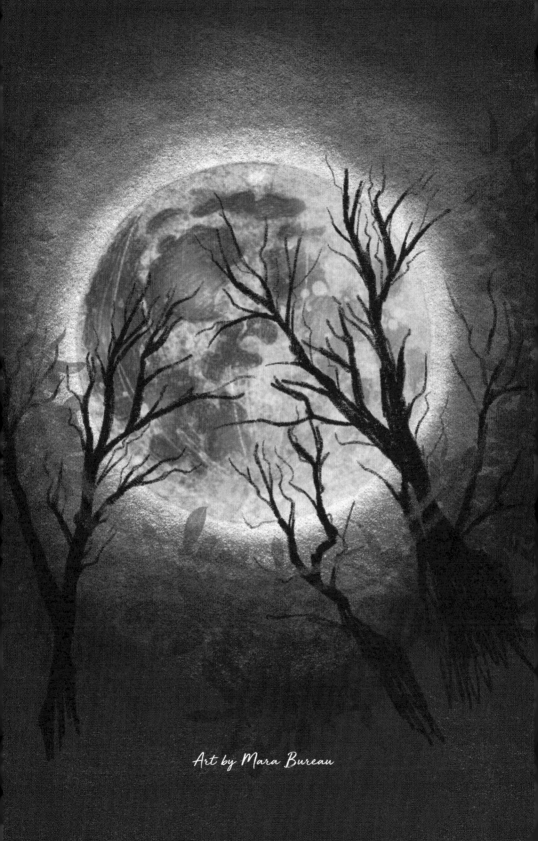

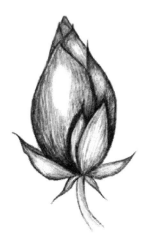

There are three things that are givens about labor: It's hard work, it hurts a lot, and you can do it. That's the bottom line. All the rest you learn is icing on the cake.

—Pam England and Rob Horowitz,
Birthing from Within

Riding a Tsunami

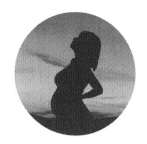

by Janelle Connor
Oakfield, Nova Scotia
Third-Place 2019

July 14th, 2016, was the most physically, emotionally, and mentally gruelling day of my life. The day I tested my capacity for coping with discomfort – the agony, the convulsions, and the fear. The day I travelled out of body when I reached the absolute peak and limit of my endurance.

I would do it all over again. The same choices, mistakes, and obstacles. Again and again, but with more confidence...

... because it was also the day I realized pure, unconditional, radiant love. The day I gained access to my greatest source of pride and happiness. The day I uncovered a next-level appreciation and respect for every mother on this planet.

It was the day our charismatic, playful, sensitive, daring, and wildly entertaining son was born. The day my life turned a new chapter, and I became part of a much bigger story. The day I stepped into motherhood and became "Kai's mom."

Monday, July 11th, after a night of restless sleep from hip pain and vivid dreams, we drove to our midwife's office. We sipped tea and chatted briefly about how I was feeling. I explained I was anxious and ready to get things started. You know, the usual 40-week thought process of "let's get this baby out of me."

We went ahead and did the stretch and sweep. The midwife was shocked to discover I was already 4 cm dilated and 80% effaced.

She looked at us and she said, "You will be meeting your son in less than 48 hours!"

Even with days' worth of Braxton Hicks contractions and false labour starts, we were still in shock to hear this news. We felt excited, relieved, but also slightly panicked.

Almost an hour after the sweep, I started to time contractions five minutes apart. They were painful but manageable (this is the part you see in the movies).

When we arrived back at home, I tried everything to relax and get comfortable. However, as the day went on, my contractions picked up in intensity and lasted all night.

This was the challenging part about early labour; it can be extremely long.

I was up all night with contractions and knew I wasn't giving my body the rest it needed. Despite my discomfort, I knew it wasn't active labour because the contractions were not progressing.

By 10 a.m., I reached a breaking point and called the midwife for support. She came to the house to check my cervix and confirmed I was 5 cm.

Although my 1 cm progression seemed insignificant, my midwife assured me this was great progress. Hearing her excitement made me also celebrate my success. *I made it this far on my own in the comfort of our home. Maybe I can do this*, I thought.

Our midwife instructed us to stay at home as long as possible and reminded us that if we were in active labour, the contractions would not stop with rest. I took her advice for a few hours, but by 4 p.m., I was completely drained and not even the thought of meeting our son could keep me going.

We packed up the vehicle and headed to the hospital. Apart of me just needed reassurance that we were progressing. I was done with guessing.

At this point, I had not slept in two days so naturally, my mind started to play tricks on me. Once I arrived at the hospital, my contractions stalled. My body was undoubtedly adjusting to the new bright and sterile atmosphere. My midwife explained that if you perceive danger, your body will protect the baby by stalling labour.

Once my contractions were measurable again, the nurse came in to check.

"You are 5 cm," she said. I instantly started to cry; I was so discouraged.

The nurse looked at me sympathetically and asked, "Would you like something to help you sleep, my dear?"

I sat straight up in the bed and said, "Yes, please!"

The nurse mixed up a sleep cocktail of morphine and Gravol, and I drifted into a blissful sleep. I woke up around 1 a.m. to my husband staring at me as if I just returned to Earth. He wasn't wrong – it was a wonderful escape.

We were discharged from the hospital so we could go home and get more rest.

Wednesday, July 13th, I woke up from the second half of the greatest sleep of my life. I started my day feeling less anxious with a new attitude. Suddenly, I didn't mind still being pregnant. Sleep is a powerful thing.

Jer and I decided to make the most of the beautiful summer day. We took a long and slow walk at a park near our house and sat next to the lake. Being around water was calming and helped take my mind off the contractions.

I previously lost my appetite in the week leading up to this day, but suddenly, I felt an overwhelming desire to consume a large number of calories. When we got home from the park, I took a bath to relax. I decided to stop putting pressure on myself to time contractions and just let them come and go. I trusted my body would tell me if it was the real deal.

I went to bed that night in a calm state. In fact, I felt so comfortable, I took the mattress protector off our bed because it was bunching up and driving me crazy. I figured if I was going into labour at this stage, it wouldn't involve my water breaking.

Boy, was I ever wrong! Maybe I was in denial.

Thursday, July 14th, sometime around midnight, my water broke in a *major* way. It was like popping a huge water balloon and this sudden gush of water made me jump out of bed. I walked to the bathroom as amniotic fluid leaked out of me like a faucet onto our hardwood floors. All I could think was, *this is it! We will finally meet our son!*

That thought was immediately followed by the logical planner in me going through my hospital checklist. Maybe I should have a bath, pack snacks, call my mom, straighten my hair… But these thoughts were abruptly interrupted by a powerful sensation that took me to my knees.

As soon as the contraction was over, I woke Jer up in the most dramatic way possible.

I shouted, "My water broke, and we need to go to the hospital right now!" Jer opened his eyes and looked around. "Hmm, is that fluid on the bed? But didn't you take the mattress cover off?"

Before I could respond, another contraction hit, and I let out a little scream and fell to my knees again. Once Jer realized the severity of the situation, he jumped out of bed. There was no need to time contractions. We just knew this was it.

Jer started the vehicle, and we left the house in less than five minutes. The entire drive to the hospital was excruciating. As I remained curled in the fetal position, terrified I would give birth in a vehicle, I repeated to myself, *it is not safe to have a baby here, it is not safe to have a baby here.* My mind was the only tool I had. I knew if I could control my thoughts, then I would be okay.

Jeremy blew through every red light going as fast as possible. He pulled next to the registration doors and ran inside to grab a wheelchair.

During registration, I remember the look on the woman's face as Jer and I lost our ability to speak. There was no health card. No signing of documents. No names provided. It was just an immediate, "Let's take you guys upstairs to the labour and delivery for assessment."

The nurse we met on the labour and delivery floor was not the warm and motherly type I was hoping for. She gave a quick and judgmental assessment with a cold glance and asked if this was my first child.

Jer responded with the obvious answer, and she replied, "Well, let me put you guys in this room and when a nurse is free, she will stop by to see how far along you actually are."

Even though I was in a wheelchair and lost complete control over my body, my mind was still very much intact. I thought about how unfair she was. Couldn't she see my body convulsing?

I went to speak but nothing came out. I was in too much pain.

Jer immediately began to advocate for me saying, "No, you need to contact our midwife and put us in a delivery room. This is the real thing; the baby is coming."

I was a little surprised by his forwardness, but it came at just the right time because I knew we were getting close.

The nurse rolled her eyes, but she did follow his orders and moved us into a delivery room. As soon as I was lifted out of the wheelchair and onto a bed, my body curled into a ball so tight that the nurse wasn't able to check for dilation. The pain was so intense, my entire body was shaking violently.

As I felt myself losing control, the nurse asked me again, "Jennifer, I need to check to see how many centimetres you are dilated."

Wait, who is Jennifer? Then, I realized Jer and I didn't register, and no one had my information.

Then a new nurse walked in, and she was a heavenly being. She had long blonde hair, blue eyes, and spoke softly as she immediately started tending to my needs. Within a few minutes, our midwife arrived, and my body was able to relax enough so she could check me.

"6 cm!" she cheered.

My mind returned to a place of panic. *All of that for just 1 cm?* I started to doubt having the courage and strength to survive natural labour. The fear of not knowing how long the pain would continue, or how intense it would become, trumped any confidence I had. I looked to my midwife, desperate for relief.

In that moment, I wanted every single drug available. I didn't care about my birth plan.

Although my midwife knew how badly I wanted to follow through with the birth plan, she didn't push it. Instead, she offered words of encouragement; "It is okay to take the drugs, Janelle. It doesn't mean you failed. You should be so proud with how far you've made it on your own."

She called the anesthesiologist and put in the epidural request. Just knowing help was on the way caused a massive release in my body. As soon as she hung up the phone, I had an overwhelming feeling that I needed to push. *Now.*

There was nothing stopping this urge, absolutely nothing. I could have been in the middle of a busy intersection and not been able to stall this freight train racing through my body.

My midwife did a quick check, and I was 10 cm dilated. My transition, the final phase of labour, from 6 cm to 10 cm, was a brief (yet enduring) two minutes.

Everyone around me started moving quickly. At this point, I still had on the shirt I wore to hospital; I guess no time for johnny shirts or cute birthing robes. They quickly set up equipment and moved tables around.

This was when my midwife came over to deliver the news; it was too late for drugs.

She offered nitrous oxide or laughing gas to help with the pain. I put the cold plastic tube in my mouth and took a few breaths. I quickly realized I hated the taste and couldn't spare an ounce of energy to focus on breathing from a tube.

Pushing was the most challenging, yet such an incredible relief. In between pushing, I was able to experience a glorious 10 to 20 seconds of solace. During this time, Jer would bring me water, put a cold cloth on my forehead, and offer words of encouragement. In those seconds, you feel like a normal human. The pain is temporarily a memory and you're able to rest and recover.

The second my break was over, I found myself on another tsunami wave, carried by its surge and launched into agony and discomfort. My body took over; it knew exactly what to do.

While my body was working overtime, my mind felt oddly calm. I can only describe it as a disembodied state of being. At one point, I distinctively remember the feeling that I was looking down at the entire room watching the whole thing.

I saw Jer whisper to our midwife, "Her face is really red. Is she going to be okay?"

My midwife smiled and said, "Your wife is in labour. This is very normal."

My altered state of consciousness encouraged me to stay grounded and I felt instructed to access my power within. As I continued to surrender, I witnessed strength and endurance I didn't know I possessed. I listened to my instincts and allowed my body to guide me. With each push, I could feel the sensation, relief, and satisfaction of my son in my arms. It was the only motivation I needed.

When my midwife told me she could see his head full of brown hair, I nearly died of joy. It took a few more strenuous pushes and then suddenly, I could hear him crying. The midwife carefully laid him on my chest and the tsunami intensity of the waves, the fear, the pain, everything melted away. I slipped into a state of pure bliss. I was in absolute awe of this life force we created.

I really can't account for what took place in the delivery room after Kai was in my arms. However, there is a bit of magic to this story I need to share – something I could never forget.

After Kai was safely in my arms with the room still buzzing with activity, something caught my eye in the window. It was around 3 a.m. and completely dark out but I could sense a presence. My eyes were directed to the window, and I saw a figure sitting on its ledge. I looked a little closer and realized it was a dove. I instantly got chills all over my body. Was I hallucinating?

I needed validation. Was this really a dove or was I dreaming?

I reached for the angelic nurse and said, "Excuse me, is that a dove in the window?"

She looked down at me, confused, before looking over her shoulder. "Wow! Yes, a dove." She paused. "Very unusual."

I am glad she witnessed it along with Jer, so I can tell this story without questioning whether it was real or an illusion. Reflecting, I didn't need testament from my nurse. I am allowed to hold my own suspicions of this dove, and why it chose to sit on my delivery room window at the exact moment of Kai's arrival.

Kai entering this world was truly a transformational experience. It was the day I learned to surrender and release and the day I witnessed an inner intelligence guide me through labour. A hard-wired deep knowledge moved and flowed through my body on autopilot.

Leaving the hospital the next day, I walked out with a new identity, a sureness that wasn't there before. Labour undoubtedly gave me a crash course in confidence. I was now fully aware of just how daring, tenacious, and resilient I could be, and this will stay with me till I die.

For all the soon-to-be mamas reading along, here is an insider tip: you have a will and determination made of titanium inside of you. Please don't question, doubt, or underestimate this strength.

Rest assured, there is a grit and badassery lying dormant that will wake at just the right moment. Please trust in this.

About Janelle

Janelle Connor is from Oakfield, Nova Scotia. She is a wife, student, financial advisor, aspiring writer, and a proud mama to a curious and charismatic little boy. To read more from Janelle, visit her blog at https://soulnourished.home.blog/

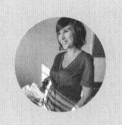

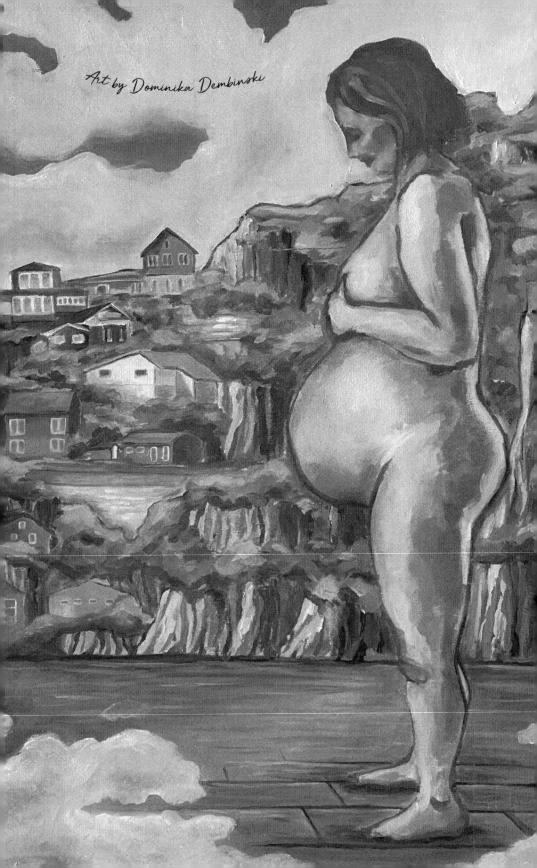

It All Makes Sense Now

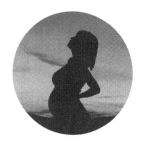

by Camille Ramsperger
Keswick, Ontario

Before having my baby, I wasn't sure I even wanted kids. I didn't know if I would ever be ready or if I would even make a good mother.

When I was pregnant, it was so difficult. I couldn't understand how anyone could go through with pregnancy more than once, *willingly*, when they knew what it was like.

This is the story of how my boy came into the world and changed my whole life forever.

"Quiet, shy, reserved..." I'm going to say quiet again, because I can't emphasize that enough.

That was my mother's immediate answer when I asked her to describe me. Not exactly the answer any employer would be looking for during an interview, but perfectly accurate to describe my personality otherwise.

Or so I thought.

Going through labour and birth brought out a side of me that not only surprised myself, but also everyone who had the pleasure of having their eardrums pop in my presence.

Let's have a brief throwback to how this all started. When I found out I was pregnant, after the initial state of shock, reality set in that if I went through with this, I would be a single mother to a child. A real, human child. I didn't tell anyone for weeks, going back and forth in my head about what I wanted to do. Realistically, this was some sort of formality I was forcing myself to endure, as I knew exactly what I would end up choosing.

So, there I was, nine months later, about to have the most perfect baby boy. Not that I knew that at the time. This pregnancy was a surprise to start with. I figured everything might as well remain a surprise through to the very end (even though I *knew* he would be a boy. Mother's intuition, I suppose).

It was already the longest day of the year when 2 o'clock in the morning came around for the second time and I felt cramping in my lower abdomen and back. Little did I know, the next nine hours would make the day feel even longer.

Not to panic, I told myself, *this is your first baby.* There is no way you're going into labour a day early. It's probably just Braxton Hicks. Ha! Let's all laugh together now at how much denial I was in at the time.

I barely had time to adjust to the thought that my baby was coming than the contractions were already five minutes apart. My mom heard me walking around and woke up, coming to see what I was doing. "I think I'm in labour."

You should know that I was like the boy who cried wolf during the later stages of my pregnancy. At least a dozen times in the last few weeks, I had fooled my mom into thinking I was in labour by stopping mid-track and saying, "Oof, I think that was a contraction," while grabbing my rounded belly, watching her face turn to a mixture of fear and excitement, only to say, "Just kidding," and watch her face fall with slight annoyance and disappointment. She was almost more excited for this baby than I was. Almost.

When I didn't follow through with my regular joking remarks, I could feel her excitement rising.

"We're about to meet this baby," she said, giddiness apparent in her voice.

The contractions continued, closer and closer together. They were excruciating. I was screaming and holding back tears. I remember my mother and my sister beside me while I was in the tub trying to relax telling me, "This isn't the worst part yet," which, as you can imagine, did not help put me at ease.

Having gone through pregnancy without a partner, I knew I wanted to have this baby by myself. I wanted everyone out of the room when it was time to push so that in that first moment when he would be in my arms, it would just be the two of us, as it had been for the past nine months. But I did agree that my mother and sister could be in the room as long as it wasn't yet time to push. I am eternally thankful for their presence. They held my hands, pushed on my hips to relieve some pressure, brought me ice packs, sips of water and small bites of food (which I immediately vomited, but the sentiment was appreciated nonetheless), and continuously offered words of encouragement. I knew I could do this, because I had these two amazing women by my side who I love and who had been through pregnancies themselves. I trusted them.

I was adamant about giving birth at home, in the comfort of my own bedroom, surrounded by familiar things. I wanted to have my baby in my arms, and not have to eventually get into a car to go home once the baby was here. I wanted to be home already. My midwife had told me prior to all of this that if I changed my mind and wanted to go to the hospital, all I had to do was say it and it would all be arranged for me. I shrugged that off.

"Pfft," I said, "I can handle it. No matter how much it hurts, this baby has to come out, so might as well go through with it at home."

"Well, just in case, remember that you do have that option. You just say the word."

And that was that. I pushed that thought to the back of my mind, because to me, that wasn't an option. I knew what I wanted, albeit there were many contractions that made me want to change my mind. Every scream I let out, I made sure not to state any desire to go to the hospital.

Back to my labour, the contractions were five minutes apart, and when the midwife got there around 5:30 a.m., I was already at 7 cm dilated.

"Thank God, that means it's almost time to push," I naively said.

I could see the midwife and my family glancing at each other with uneasy looks on their faces. No one wanted to tell me that progressing to seven centimetres that fast does not mean the last three centimetres would be equally fast. They didn't have to tell me; I saw their faces. I understood what they did not say, and my heart sank. This was going to hurt.

And it did, it really did.

The next few hours were a bit of a blur. There are, however, several moments that I won't soon forget. My baby's head was turned in the wrong direction, and so the midwife had me stand and sit and squat in numerous positions during contractions to try to turn him. I remember this vividly because I just wanted to cry and scream out and curl into a ball, which was the least uncomfortable. The lesser of all evil positions.

For one contraction, I had my right leg up on a chair. For the next, my left leg. Then, I had to sit on the toilet and have a contraction there. Then, I had to stand. Then, I put my legs back on the chair. I was still screaming. It was debilitating, but it worked because, when she checked me next, his head had turned, and I was at 9 cm. What a relief. Now I knew we were getting close and I was getting the urge to push.

I don't know what it's like for all women who go through labour, but when I had the urge to push and was told I couldn't, it was very, *very* difficult not to. My body and mind were barely working together in that moment. It took a lot of willpower to convince myself not to push. My midwife was advising me not to push until I got to 10 cm, or I might damage and enflame the birth canal, making it even more difficult to push the baby out. I could understand that, but my muscles just weren't listening. Somehow, I made it to 10 cm without too much damage, and it was just about time to meet my son.

I pushed for nearly an hour, then the midwife told me she could see his head. I looked down and I thought it was a bum. The bony plates in my baby's head that would later fuse together were overlapped on top of each other and looked like a little baby bottom. He had a decent amount of hair when he was born, so I knew it was his head, but this gave me slight comedic relief in a time of immense pain.

His head was out. My contraction ended. It took nearly two minutes for my next contraction to start again so I could continue pushing, but in the meantime, I was admiring this perfect little skull, that I loved so much already, hanging out of my hoo-hah. Some more comedic relief. In hindsight, it must have been pretty strange, but in the moment, I was awestruck. What a perfect little head. It took a fraction of a push for the rest of his body to come out, and he was then laid onto my chest and covered with a blanket.

I looked into his dark brown eyes, and I could feel my own start to water. This is my baby. *My* baby. He's here, and he's mine. I lifted the blanket briefly to confirm what I already knew. He's perfect. I still, to this day, don't believe that something so perfect came out of me.

In the background, my midwife was telling me that I needed stitches, and that it would sting a bit, and I could not have cared less. I had my baby in my arms, and that is all I could focus on.

Every ounce of pain I had felt, not only in labour but throughout my entire pregnancy, was worth it and already forgotten about. I would go through it a hundred million gazillion times for this little boy, and he would be worth it every time.

I don't know what I pictured before I went into labour. I don't really know if I pictured anything or expected anything. I had never been through it before, so I wasn't sure how it would all play out. What I can say, though, is that everything that happened was aligned exactly with what I would have hoped for. A home birth with the support of two wonderful women during labour and giving birth on my own with only the assistance of the midwives as I wished for, to meet my son for the first time, a perfect, healthy little baby boy to call my own.

Before having my baby, I wasn't sure I even wanted kids. Now that I have my sweet little baby boy in my arms, I don't know how women ever stop.

About Camille

Camille Ramsperger is a 26-year-old single mother to a beautiful baby boy named Theodore. She is a full-time nurse working in the emergency department at her nearest hospital. She meant to write her birth story so as not to forget it, and the Birth Story Contest gave her the motivation to do so.

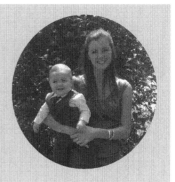

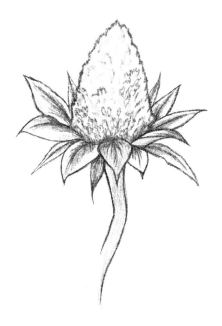

If you ask a random stranger, 'Who is the legal authority in the labor and delivery room?' many people might say, 'the doctor.' Although the doctor is viewed as an authority figure by many people, he or she is not the legal authority over the woman's body or baby. The person who is giving birth is the one who has right to say 'yes' or 'no' to any medical care offered to them.

—**Rebecca Dekker,** *Babies Are Not Pizzas: They're Born, Not Delivered.*

Worth It

by Angela Douglas
Summerland, British Columbia

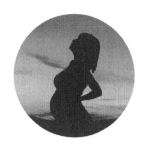

I will start this story by saying my son was perfect. Unscathed, unharmed, and a 9 on the Apgar scale. His birth was not perfect. It was traumatic. Not so much so that it stopped me from doing it again. I gave birth to another happy, healthy child 19 months later, and her birth was wonderful. I had a midwife the second time, which made all the difference in the world.

The pregnancy was a planned surprise. I was diagnosed with Polycystic Ovary Syndrome (PCOS) three months prior and was in a brand-new relationship. As new as it was, we knew where we wanted the future to go, and that we didn't have time to waste. We tried from early on.

When I found out I was pregnant, I was shocked and elated. I didn't think it would happen at all, let alone so quickly. We had only been together for 11 weeks at this point.

The pregnancy started off well. Brutal morning sickness, but I managed. Cravings that started off normal and got weird fast.

We got married in Vegas (and are still married today), so we could have a quick and affordable union, and all have the same last name. A few weeks after we got back, I really popped. Shortly after, that I started swelling and having a hard time getting around. I couldn't explain what the problem was until I was diagnosed with high blood pressure, and then pre-eclampsia.

By the time I was 26 weeks pregnant, I had to have weekly stress tests in the hospital; they checked the protein in my urine, heartbeat of the baby, blood pressure, etc. At 32 weeks, I was told to go on bed rest, and I made it to 38 weeks.

I was getting ready for my 38-week appointment, and I was just going to sludge out the door as is, in the only item of maternity clothing that still fit. At this point, I had gained close to 100 pounds. Something inside me said I had better have a shower in case this was it. My proteins had been increasing at the last few appointments, and at this point, I was feeling extremely unwell. My face and eyes were swollen, my legs were like tree trunks, and the swelling was causing them to itch.

"Every day inside is a gift," my doctor told me over and over. If I can just make it to 38 weeks, my son would be fully developed.

I had a long shower, and headed out the door, with one last look around my apartment, wondering if that was the last time I would ever be alone.

I was right. I provided my urine sample and met with Grover (my doctor). He had a kind and informal style, sitting on top of his desk swinging his legs like a child. I liked it. He delivered tough news in an easy manner. "Well, Angela," he said. "It's time. Time to go across the street and induce this baby."

Okay, I wasn't fully expecting that. I thought they would set an appointment time, or something where I could give my husband and sister a heads up. Maybe whip home and grab my hospital bag. But no. It was a no.

"Your proteins are high, and your blood pressure is very high. You have preeclampsia, and you need to evict your tenant for both of your health. You made it to 38 weeks, you should be very proud."

Normally, I protest everything he says. I take a long time to digest information, I throw up little problems, and discuss details that don't matter. All I could do was nod.

It wasn't until I was moving my car across the street that it sunk in. I called my husband and got his voicemail. He was at the scene of a five-alarm fire. "Hey, hun, just me, proteins are high, preeclampsia is bad, I am at the hospital being induced. Bye."

Then another stellar, detail-filled phone call to my sister that said much the same, only I added that I hope they don't tow my car when the meter runs out.

Eventually, they both arrived, my car was handled, and the hospital bag was brought in. I had been induced with the gel. All the gel did was make me feel like I had to have a bowel movement for the next 20 hours, and it caused period-like cramps. I was checked a handful of times and no dilation was happening. Throughout those 20 hours, I was given the gel twice more, and was eventually given a Pitocin drip.

The next step was to break my water. I was already exhausted. I hadn't slept the night before going into the hospital, and I sure as heck didn't sleep during cramp-gate either. I was tired and hungry. They weren't letting me eat, which I later learned, was in case I needed surgery.

Things were not moving along, I was wrecked, and still had to deliver a child. I was given the option to have an epidural with the water break. I took it.

I had given these specific instructions to family and friends: "I only want my husband and my sister at the hospital during the birth." Somehow, my mom (who lives far away) was in the lobby, and right during the middle of my legs-wide-open-getting-my-water-broken moment, my clueless father-in-law and his wife (who also live far away) waltzed into the room. I was mortified, and they were oblivious. I shot my husband a look and he quickly ushered them out of the room.

Fast forward an hour or so and labour is ticking along according to the machines I was hooked up to and my latest dilation check. This was great, except the epidural wasn't working on one side. I could feel labour pains but only on that side of my body. After more than an hour of that torture, the anesthesiologist came back in and attempted a second epidural.

The epidural kicked in and worked, thank goodness, and I fell asleep. Hard. I was snoring my face off when, in my dream, I could feel a major pressure down there, like something was coming out. I woke up and felt the pressure again. I looked over to the nurse who had been assigned to monitor me around the clock and said, "I think the head is out."

She smiled and said, "Oh I don't think so, sweetie. It's your first baby and…" as she lifted the sheet to check, her face changed and so did her tone. "Yep, heads almost there. I'm going to go grab the doctor now," and away she ran.

The doctor came in, one from the team of doctors I was assigned to but had never met. From the first push to the last, it was only about 20 minutes. Not bad for a first baby, I kept hearing.

I reached down and grabbed my boy from them as he came out. He looked perfect. He was big, and chubby, and well developed. His eyes were open, and he was alert, looking right at me and then all around the room. He was breathing, but he wasn't crying. It was so quiet, stoic, and magical. I held him for a few minutes in awe.

The doctors were having a hard time delivering the placenta, and I was trying to push but nothing was happening. They said I needed to have a manual removal performed or to have surgery. They warned that they would not be able to top up the epidural, as I had already had "too much," and the epidural was too high to help for this purpose anyway. The manual procedure consisted of something that belongs in a barnyard. I chose to do it anyway, because I didn't want to have the surgery. A female doctor then entered the room. They chose her to do the procedure because her arms were slimmer and longer. I still shudder at the memory.

Without detail, she attempted more than once. It was painful, and I started feeling weak. I looked at my beautiful baby, looking right at me, and didn't notice the chaos around me. Everything was beeping and flashing, and people were coming in and out. At some point, I looked at my mom who had entered the room to see us. I could see her tearing up at the sight of her first grandchild, and then I saw fear in her eyes. I saw others with the same expression. Then, I started to feel faint. I was hemorrhaging and my family was witnessing it all.

I was rushed into surgery, unconscious. I came to in a surgery room with bright lights shining down on me. I was signing something I couldn't see. I was convulsing so much that one person was holding the clipboard with the form and someone else was holding my hand with the pen in it. Everything went dark.

Five hours later, I woke up in post-op. I couldn't talk because my throat hurt, and the nurses didn't know I was awake because my eyes were so swollen that you couldn't tell if they were open or not. Eventually, I got their attention and begged them to take me to my family. They wheeled me up the stairs and spoke to me casually, as though I had been in there for a haircut. No info about my surgery, just a ride upstairs.

Nothing else mattered when I entered that room. My husband was holding my son almost asleep with his finger in his mouth. My baby must have been so hungry. My mom and sister were still there. They all waited until they saw me. They were given no updates. I got some big hugs before they left to catch up on some overdue sleep.

My husband's dad and wife showed up unannounced again. They insisted on holding the baby and posing for pictures without realizing what we had just been through, or that I hadn't held my own son yet, except for that brief moment at birth. I whispered expletives in my husband's ear. Minutes later, they were gone. All of them. They were hungry and wanted to eat, so I told hubby to go ahead with them. Get some food, get some rest, I would be fine. I am fine.

I wasn't fine at all, but I wanted to be alone. I held my Johnny and promised him I would never leave him like that again. I bawled like a newborn, which was ironic, because he didn't.

We spent the next five days in the hospital, the next two weeks recovering from a major infection likely due to the procedure, and endured subsequent surgeries and pain as a result. I also suffered from postpartum depression.

It was all worth it. I have this wonderful human being in my life. It took me years to be able to talk about this. In fact, I just read the hospital records earlier this year, to try to fill some holes and get closure. I almost died, and now know my son's life was at risk as well, with the preeclampsia and undiagnosed placenta accreta.

I almost died, but I didn't. I was terrified to have another child, but I did. I survived and love my life to pieces. I wouldn't change anything now, but

I may have gone back in time and found a midwife or a doula to advocate for me. I was so vulnerable during this time in my life. I had no voice until now. Thank you for reading.

About Angela

Angela Douglas is a marketing communications professional, author, and proud mother. She writes thrillers and non-fiction. This story marked her return to writing after a lengthy absence. When she isn't working, she writes in her studio with her bulldog Frankie. Angela's debut psychological thriller *EVERY FALL*, comes out in January 2025. Angela lives in the Okanagan with her husband and kids.

Find Angela at https://www.angeladouglas.ca or @anglynndouglas on social media.

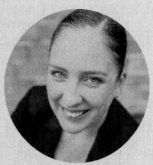

Birth Plan

by Brittany Oliver
Welland, Ontario

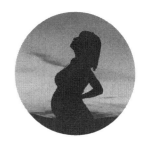

I was longingly planning a home birth in the loving, capable hands of one of my best friends who is also a midwife at my clinic. I did a local hypno-birthing class to prepare myself for labour and every night I visualized that straightforward, normal (but intense) vaginal birth in my bed surrounded by my amazing husband and mother.

Unfortunately, I ended up with prodromal early labour and then dystocia at 4 cm, despite artificial rupture of membranes at home. I transferred in for epidural and oxytocin augment, but the interventions were unsuccessful, and I was still 4 cm. My care team and I decided it was time for a C-section.

Although the surgery went smoothly, I really struggled with how my birth ended up. Of course, I was grateful and over the moon to finally meet my healthy girl (who was 11 days past due), but I grieved my home birth and vaginal delivery. I wrote this poem to help process my feelings and the bizarre presence of conflicting sadness in a time of such happiness. I truly hope it serves to normalize any similar feelings for anyone else who reads it.

Birth Plan

You were supposed to be born at home
Your perfect head through feminine flora
Into the sheets we anxiously and excitedly prepared
Into the room where we first dreamt of your existence
Into the loving hands of my midwife
How many times had I envisioned that moment?
Nature bringing me to the very edge

but safe, supported and warm in my bed
I cherished that moment in my mind, nurtured it
Your cry, my cry, your wet tiny body being gracefully lifted onto my stomach
Your old home deflated beneath you
My hands providing immediate comfort in your new surroundings

How I longed for it
To feel powerful, primal, out of control even
I craved it
The messiness, the rawness
I wanted to reach for you right away, absent of thought – led only by emotion
A memory to treasure within these familiar walls

But my story, although unique and beautiful…
Left me defeated.
Left me yearning.
Left me with a scar.

Questions reeled through my mind,
irrational, absurd but impossible to silence.
Am I not worthy enough?
Am I not wilful enough?
Am I not woman enough?

Gratefulness and grief teetered within me the day
I brought you home
You had always belonged there
Love instantly swelled within its walls
Hopes, dreams and visions of the future whizzed around corners and
  through doorways
My baby was home
But my heart still ached

BIRTH PLAN

The home birth gear was piled in the corner
of the bedroom
Ready, eager and totally useless.

Sudden loss and emptiness
I swat away the sorrow
It doesn't feel welcome
I should be elated
And I am confused because I am

But I hadn't visualized the sterility, bright lights
 and smell of cautery
My stomach, once a beautiful temple of life
was numb and disinfected
I never dreamt I would hear your first cry
behind a wall of blue
My hands unable to reach for you, my baby
Yet in that moment I was transformed
I was a mother
And the happiness and bliss I felt was immense
You were here.
The journey long and painful
in many ways
But you were here
And you my dear, you are perfect
Just as I suspected
And I would do it all again a thousand times over

So, I will wear my scar proudly
Every time I let out a good belly laugh it will dance
Every time I follow my gut it will be my arrow
Every time I pull you close it will be there – the embrace of our
   inseparable time together

I still ache

I don't know why things went the way they did

There were no clear answers

Perhaps my heart couldn't bear to let you distance yourself any further;

my body refusing to accept your impending absence,

my womb gripping its greatest creation.

All I know is that we had to create a path for you where none existed

And that in and of itself is kind of poetic

You will always find a way

My pioneer, my trailblazer.

My baby.

About Brittany

Brittany Oliver has been a midwife for over five years. She loves connecting with clients, catching babies and story-telling. Her goal is to continue sharing her creative works in hopes to bring more love and empathy and laughter to the world. Brittany lives in the Niagara region of Ontario with her husband and young daughter.

Instagram Page: @wit.by.brit

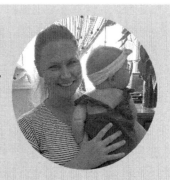

Delivered

by Christine Folan
Chatham, Ontario

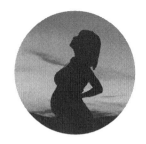

Although I did not use a midwife or doula for the birth of my children, I feel that I have a story that can resonate with mothers who have been judged or discriminated against since their children were born via caesarean section. I also feel as though young or inexperienced mothers may be able to relate to my story since my first childbirth was somewhat traumatic, caused in part by my own lack of knowledge and affirmation.

I had never questioned or truly reflected upon the Hollywood representation of labour and childbirth until my own son was born. Why would I ever have reason to doubt that the breaking of a woman's water would signal immediate and powerful contractions? Why would I have reason to wonder whether it was realistic for women to push for five minutes, only to successfully deliver a clean(ish), plump, and gurgling baby?

When I finally delivered my son, he was skinny. He was blue. He was quiet.

My story is a happy one. Doctors and nurses quickly worked to revive my baby while my husband looked on, feigning an easy and casual expression, even when I managed to get myself together long enough to ask him why the baby wasn't crying. I had been huffing gas like it was oxygen and had been in active labour for almost 12 hours. I was strapped to a surgical table, hands out to my sides, and my insides out to the world. My husband told me they hadn't yet removed my baby. I believed him and allowed myself to fall back into the cloud of medicinal haze and unconsciousness.

I am not a petite woman. I have no ass to speak of, a trait that both of my children seem to have inherited, but one would never suspect that labour and childbirth would not be possible for my body. I have hips. I have large breasts. I look like a baby maker.

Then, my body refused to cooperate, and my child almost died inside of me. While my husband struggled at my side to keep his composure and to keep me calm, I couldn't help but picture those women I had seen on television and in films. They would stop suddenly, mid-sentence, and then look down comically. The camera would follow their gaze to a tiny, neat puddle on the floor between immaculate, white sneakers. The mother would then be held under her arms while she waddled to a wheelchair or to the backseat of a car, only to be delivered of her baby moments later. My contractions began 72 hours before my baby was delivered. No cute puddle for me. It would come hours later while I struggled on a hospital bed, arms straining and pulling against the metal bed rails as I pushed.

My husband and I were sent home from the hospital twice before we were finally admitted. I should have fought. I should have advocated for myself. Instead, I thought of those ridiculous and screaming women from television and thought to myself, "It's fine. I can do this. I'm strong."

Twenty-four hours after my contractions began and after being sent home twice, I vomited in my bathtub from the pain. My mother helped to clean me up and washed my hair like she did when I was a child. My husband drove me to my OB/GYN, who gave me a shot of morphine and then sent me home to get some sleep. I hadn't even begun to dilate. Finally, roughly 48 hours after contractions had begun, I was admitted to the hospital, where I traded my sweat-soaked maternity clothes for the rough blue cloth of a hospital gown.

After four hours of pushing, I repeated, "I can do this. I'm strong," when the doctor who assisted my delivery had me sign a waiver that would allow him to use forceps and protect him should anything go wrong. My signature contained mostly legible letters.

After more unsuccessful pushing, another waiver. An emergency caesarean section.

My signature consisted of an uppercase letter followed by a wave. My hand was shaking so badly that I could barely hold the pen.

The anaesthesiologist on call was away and had to be summoned. More waiting. My doctor leaned in and told me to stop pushing while we waited. My body, no longer my own, kept up its frantic rhythm of contract and push without my allocation or provocation. I'd been sucking down a gas that would, according to my nurse, help to alleviate the discomfort. I couldn't tell you its name to save my life. I was exhausted. I was just as much in the audience as I had been at home on my couch, watching thin women with beautifully curled hair bring forth their babies on TV. My hair was stringy. I didn't wash it for another three days.

I made small talk with a nurse who sat at my side during the procedure. I knew her mother. My mind rejoiced at the change of subject. The doctor went to work and quickly, I felt the change in pressure, the sudden and visceral empty that overcame me when my son was lifted from my body. But the silence was wrong. Babies always cried immediately after delivery. They were brought, fat and suckling, to their mothers. My baby, the weight that had been living beneath my ribs for the past nine months, was suddenly gone. Only he didn't appear at my breast like some cherubic apparition. He was taken away somewhere. My husband mentioned that he was curious and would follow the baby. It wasn't until a few days had passed that he admitted that he had seen our son's blue and limp body but hadn't wanted to alarm me.

I continued chatting with my nurse about her mother while he was resuscitated.

When I think back on the birth of my son, the word that comes to mind is lucky. I was lucky. My husband was lucky. My son was lucky. The forceps had left a mark barely an inch from his left eye. His skull was bruised from the incessant pressure and beating it received from my pelvic bone.

He was quickly revived thanks to the hard work and determination of an amazing team of healthcare professionals. Not all babies are so lucky.

When they finally brought my boy to me, wrapped in a blue hospital blanket, my first thoughts were that he looked like a potato. The next thoughts were that I now had no idea what to do with this tiny human they had handed me. I didn't know him.

My faithful television and movie mothers had led me to believe that these first moments, the first time that I held my child, I would be overcome with love for him. I would cry. I would kiss his tiny face and feel my heart swell. All I felt was tired, empty, and thanks to the aforementioned gas, dazed.

The most powerful feelings I felt those first few days were fear and anxiety. Everything and anything could harm or kill my baby. Worse, I still didn't feel as though I loved him. I wanted him safe and secure, but I didn't know if I felt bonded to him. I wasn't overcome with a blinding joy, nor did I hear a crescendo of angels when I looked at his sleeping form.

What they don't tell you in television and films is that childbirth is not practical, or neat, or conducive to a well-structured plotline. It is unpredictable, it is messy, and it can be difficult to advocate for yourself since it can be so difficult to truly work out what you are feeling and experiencing. My doctor was young and new to the game, and so was I. We waded through our inexperience together and came out the other side as victors. When I was pregnant with my second child, I went back to him.

We planned my second section during one of my first prenatal visits. My husband was completely supportive of my decision since he carried his own scars and trauma from my son's birth, painful and frightening scenes that have etched themselves into a place in his mind I cannot conceive of or even really understand. I watched myself going through the steps of labour and delivery as if I were an outside observer. So did my husband, although his experience wasn't clouded by a foreign numbness as mine is whenever I try to think back on it.

While pregnant with my daughter, I allowed myself to make decisions that I had never entertained during my first pregnancy, and I refused to read or to listen to mothers (and fathers) who argued that a caesarean birth wasn't the real deal. That it didn't count.

It's the coward's way out.

It's cheating.

It's not a natural birth.

My son is alive today because he was lucky. The only thing unnatural about his birth is that his mother was such a passive participant. I hadn't really known what to expect because even though my husband and I had done the birthing class, even though our mothers had shared their own stories, even though friends had warned us as to what to expect, I had been inundated with the falsified and pretty images that flashed from my screen. These unnatural expectations had seeped themselves in so deep that they lived undetected until the moment I began my own birth story, and they swarmed to the surface. I do not regret my epidural, and I am not ashamed that I needed help managing my pain. As far as I know, my hospital does not hand out medals to women who complete their labours and deliveries without the help of drugs.

What I do regret is my passivity, that I allowed myself to become a bystander to what was happening. I do not pretend to know better than the medical professionals who helped me, but I do know my body. I knew that something was wrong with it, that it had been somehow defeated. I should have thrown the forceps waiver back into my doctor's face and screamed that he cut me open and take out my baby. But who wants to be the hysterical and screaming mother?

When my daughter was born via a planned section, I was alert. I was aware. I was prepared.

She came out screaming for the both of us.

She made sure she was heard.

About Christine

Christine Folan is a married mother of two, living in Southwestern Ontario. She is a high school English and drama teacher for the French Catholic School Board in her region. An avid reader, she is trying to instill a love of fantasy, adventure, and mystery into her children by making them lovers of books and stories.

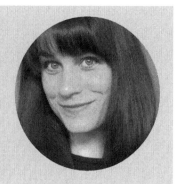

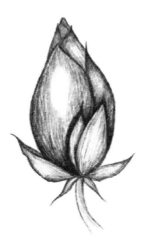

Caring for an infant is an epic commitment of the will to work in tandem with the heart, as well as the instinct.

— **Naomi Wolf,** *Misconceptions*

She Who Brings Forth the Blossoms

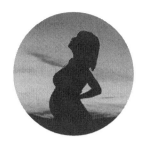

by Leah Timmermann
Maberly, Ontario

As a young sprout, I was surrounded by radiant, flourishing blooms of mother plants. They shaded me from the sun, fed and nourished me. They were my own mother, grandmothers, aunts, and neighbourhood women. I observed them in their roles and knew that I, too, desired the great privilege of becoming a mother one day. Even my young tomboy self, with the perpetually skinned knees and backwards baseball caps, couldn't deny the intense call I felt to the nurturing and womanly howl of motherhood.

A month before my 30th birthday, my partner Erik and I remarked on the speed of time. We discussed trying for a baby. After all, we joked, I was about to start a new older and wiser decade, and he, with his grey streaked hair at 34, was becoming positively geriatric. We were fortunate to become pregnant quickly.

My pregnancy progressed as the seasons changed. Leaves turned brilliant shades of amber and red. Then came the snowfall as my belly grew and grew. In Eastern Ontario, our winters can be harsh. I continued to swing a large axe, chopping wood for our stove. I had a healthy pregnancy, and my midwife helped to answer my questions and check in with me.

At holiday time, I proudly showed off my baby bump. I felt the excitement and support from my family and friends. I was asked the same questions:

"Boy or girl?" (Don't know), "When are you due?" (May), and "Aren't you scared it will hurt?", to which my answer was longer. The young sprout in me who preferred tree-forts over dolls, also held a strong belief. I was taught that women are capable and strong; that a woman with deep roots can bend and adapt to the fiercest winds.

"No, I'm not scared," I would respond. "I figure if all of us were born to mothers, and those before us, and before them, and for eons past, then I can do it too." Despite the intensity and pain that I knew awaited me, I trusted in my mind and body to rise to the occasion. I knew that if I flowed along with the ebbs and flows of labour (and of parenting, for that matter), that things would unfurl in the ways that they were meant to.

In March, I collected maple sap with my family, an annual tradition, which marks the arrival of spring. I began to waddle and grow uncomfortable. My pelvis and low back became increasingly painful. I found relief in moving my body. Fresh spring air helped calm my mind and ground me.

In April, I stopped work, and began preparing for our baby's arrival. I knit, sewed, cooked, and read. I napped, relaxed, and spoke with friends. My daily stretches and weekly trips to the pool became imperative to cope with the pelvic pain. My partner and I began nesting. We were planning a home birth and gathered our supplies, including the birth pool, the towels, and the candles. We cleaned and scrubbed, washed our bedsheets, folded newborn onesies, and put our mattress on the floor. Instead of a nursery, we planned to simplify life by having our baby live and sleep in our bedroom. Erik bought a mesh pool net from the dollar store for potential scooping in the birth tub. Spoiler alert: It was used. We met with our midwife, and asked a close friend, Danielle, to be our doula. On the last evening of April, we spoke to our precious baby and said, "We're ready to meet you!" We were so full of love and anticipation.

Mere hours later, on May 1st, I woke to irregular contractions. They were more painful than menstrual cramps, but tolerable. These sensations were completely out of the blue; I had no prior signs of early labour – no mucus plug, no bloody show. Uncertain if these were really contractions, and knowing that being a first-time mom, my labour could last for a long time, I settled into bed.

I did not sleep but I rested my body and breathed. I used my heating pad on my belly and tried to think gentle, positive thoughts. In the morning, Erik rose, and I told him that I might be in early labour. He jumped out of bed, wide-eyed, and sprang into action. We were ready and so, so excited to meet our baby.

The day carried on with more irregular contractions. I didn't time them but knew they ranged from every 3 minutes to every 15. The contractions were painful and while I could speak through them, they held my attention. I balanced rest with movement. I napped, chatted with Erik, and ate lunch. In the afternoon, we walked around our country yard. The grass was coming up and felt soft on my bare feet. I wandered over to the large magnolia tree at the edge of the property and noticed there was one, solitary pink blossom that had freshly emerged. "Imagine that," I thought. Here I was, on Mayday, May 1st, Beltane, blossoming in my own right, with the magnolia tree mirroring me – or was it the other way around?

In the evening, my contractions were about 3 to 5 minutes apart. With still no significant signs or changes, I decided to check my own cervix. I was 1 cm dilated, and with my cervix still far back (posterior) and firm. It was then that I figured I would likely be in labour for much, much longer. I had to now stop and breathe with effort through the contractions, but with my dilation, I knew I was still in early labour. I spoke on the phone with my mom, who excitedly encouraged me, and told me that she thought I was surely in labour. Erik and I made a phone call to our friends, the local Buddhist nuns. Erik and his stepfather had built the nuns a temple on their property years prior and had become close. The nuns requested we call them when I began labour, so that they could chant for us, and offer prayers of safety and love.

I cooked us a simple dinner, pausing every few minutes to breathe and lean over the side of the countertop. I obliged myself to eat but didn't have much appetite. With the sensations becoming quite painful, I drew myself a warm bath upstairs. It was nearing bedtime, and I encouraged Erik to sleep, knowing that it would likely be a long night (or weekend) of labouring.

The bath was heavenly. The warm waters enveloped me, and immediately helped to ease my aching hips and back. The contractions didn't slow down, even in the warm water, which was a good sign. I began to moan and groan with the sensations. Curious, I checked my cervix again, and was disappointed to feel that my cervix had not changed. I was still only 1 cm dilated. I then felt my first pangs of doubt. "How will I get through this?" My mind wandered to women in my life who've had lots of babies. A close friend, in particular, came to mind, who had four children vaginally. I thought about all the women around the world going through their own experiences of labour at that precise moment. I felt a deep connection to their global strength and courage.

Things then got interesting.

The contractions began to come back-to-back. I think they were about every 2 minutes apart and lasted about a minute. I held on for dear life, as the most intense pain I have ever felt surged through my body. Erik soon emerged from the bedroom. I felt good that he had come to my side, as I was beginning to need support. He brought me water to sip, and a hand to hold. With each contraction, I tried my utmost to relax my muscles and to not clench. This was hard to accomplish. The bath was still helping, but it suddenly felt cramped, the water too cold, and the surface hard on my hip bones. I asked Erik to call Danielle, our doula. I felt the need for more hands to squeeze.

No sooner had Erik left the room to make the phone call did I feel a sensation deep in my pelvis that I can only describe as feeling like two puzzle pieces clicking together. I immediately knew what I was feeling. I gingerly reached a finger inside, and confirmed that, yes, I was fully dilated, and my baby's head was right there.

"ERIIKKKKKKKKKKKKKKK!"

He called our midwife and told her things were moving along quickly. Erik asked if I wanted to move downstairs to the birthing pool. I said that I didn't think there was time to fill it up, not to mention the fact that I don't think I could have moved. It took every ounce of my focus and determination to stay present and breathe through each contraction as they barrelled through my body.

My body began pushing hard, and I fought it off, panting like a dog. I wanted our midwife and doula to be present so badly. Knowing that our baby was coming soon, I turned to Erik and yelled, "This baby is coming in 10 minutes! You better get ready." I then started barking orders about towels, and the bowl for the placenta. Erik deserved a gold medal for how incredibly calm and grounded he was, despite the exciting yet nerve-wracking scenario. He continued to hold my hand and make low, vocal sounds with me.

The midwife arrived and set up her equipment. We both felt a huge sense of calm and relief having her guiding presence and support. Within 10 minutes of her arrival, our baby's head emerged. It was a burning, fiery ring of satisfaction, as I knew my job was almost complete. Our baby's body came easily next, and she was born under water, into her father's loving hands. She was passed into my arms, and I was flooded with emotions and feelings that I will never forget. Love, gratitude, relief, and empowerment. It was after about five minutes when we realized we hadn't yet checked our baby's sex, and we cried tears of joy to discover our baby girl. My placenta came some minutes later, with a strong push. Our midwife and doula helped me waddle over to our bedroom, where we tucked into bed with our darling new little sprout. We were both fed – she from my breast, and I, chicken soup, tea, and fruit. It was now midnight, dark, and cozy in our bedroom. I felt so safe and complete.

Days later, our family and friends were eagerly awaiting to learn the baby's name. We both felt that "Maeve" would make a pretty first name. Lying happily next to her in bed, it came to me so clearly and vividly: "Maeve Magnolia." Our darling little flower girl, born on the first day of May, with the magnolia tree starting its season, with the offer of a perfect pink blossom. It was meant to be.

Becoming a mother has been a wild ride. At three months in, as I type this with one hand, as my other holds my daughter, I am happy. There are hard days, hard nights, and tears but there is also a love and connection that runs wild and deep. I often think to myself, "If I can give birth, then I can do anything." So, I have blossomed. Firstly, as a woman with strong roots and a sense of self, and now as a mother with a sense of purpose and love that I never could have imagined. So, thank you, my daughter, Maeve Magnolia; you are *she who brings forth the blossoms*.

About Leah

Leah Timmermann lives in rural Eastern Ontario. She works as a midwife but is currently on leave with her 3-month-old daughter. She and her family live in a tiny house that they built on their family's land. She loves reading, cooking, and anything outdoors.

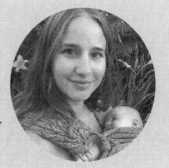

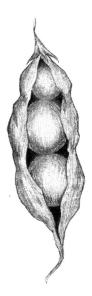

In my experience, and the findings of an ever-growing body of research, what women need in order to cope with the intensity of labour is not for the physical pain itself to be taken away. What they need instead is to feel safe.

—**Rhea Dempsey,** *Birthing with Confidence*

Our Rainbow

by Dana MacDonald
Kingston, Ontario

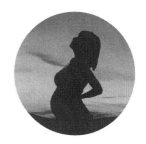

My birth story begins before a pandemic was declared, before COVID-19 became common vernacular, or masks were worn as a part of our everyday attire. It begins in September of 2018, with my first pregnancy. My partner and I were ecstatic to learn that we were expecting our first child. The pregnancy was textbook, and although the summer was incredibly hot, I had never felt more beautiful than I did carrying that child.

We did the things that new parents do; we prepped the nursery, attended birthing classes, and anxiously awaited the arrival of our future son or daughter. Unfortunately, at 37 weeks pregnant, I did not feel the baby moving as much as I normally had. I went to the doctors with a giant pit in my stomach, knowing that something did not feel right. The doctor recommended that, due to the decreased movement and my anxiety, I should have an ultrasound to make sure that everything was okay with both the baby and me. My partner decided to take time off work to meet me at the hospital and we awaited the ultrasound, as we had done so many times before. Unfortunately, this ultrasound didn't show the magic of that beautiful heart beating. Our baby was gone.

We sat in a labour and delivery room as the OB/GYN explained that they weren't sure what had happened but that the next step was to deliver. I screamed, and I sobbed, and I clutched my belly, begging it to give me some kind of movement that would tell me they had gotten this all wrong. Unfortunately, it was true, and they had to walk me through the delivery process of a stillborn. At my request, they were able to discover with the bedside ultrasound the sex of the baby. We'd have to have a name prepared and a plan in place. They told us we had lost a little boy.

The next day was spent waiting for a call to say a bed was available to deliver. My partner and I did our best to plan for an impossible day and to tell our families that their lives had changed forever as well. We went to the hospital with the mindset that we were going to make this little boy's short time with us as magical as we could, as he deserved nothing less. My partner and I played Yahtzee at the beginning of the induction, we snuggled, we cried, even managed to have a laugh or two. Dylan Thomas was born at 10:23 a.m. on September 23rd. He landed on my chest, and I was a mother. I was incredibly heartbroken but completely enamoured by the beautiful human I had carried with me for 37 weeks. The next few hours were spent staring at our beautiful boy. Our family joined us as we played music, cried, hugged, and loved that little boy with every single ounce of our bodies because we knew we didn't have much longer with him.

After a year of grieving, a year of torturous holidays and inconceivable pain, we found out we were expecting again, and our baby was due in April of 2020. Our rainbow baby was on its way, but the pregnancy wasn't quite as magical as the first. It was an anxious pregnancy. It was a pregnancy filled with fear and distrust of my own body. We were lucky to have learned that Dylan died of a true knot in his cord but there was nothing to say that this baby wouldn't succumb to the same fate or any other complication for that matter.

When the new year rolled around, we began hearing of COVID-19, as if my anxiety wasn't high enough. With that came the fear of the unknown; would my partner be able to attend the birth? What happens if I contract the virus? What happens if the baby contracts the virus? Everything was so new, and it seemed as though information was changing daily at that time. Due to the loss of our firstborn, the delivery was another induction at 37 weeks for everyone's wellbeing. As the day approached, my anxiety intensified. We arrived at the hospital to begin induction on Sunday, March 29th and although induction doesn't always follow the same path, they explained that I would likely go home and return the next day for the next step. However, this baby was telling us that he or she was ready to arrive and possibly even before the end of the day. My mind spun. The only thing I had been able to cling to was the plan set in place by the physicians. This was a wrench in my plans. We were able to go home, give our dog some kisses and cuddles, and return to the hospital with our bags and the hope that this time, we would be leaving the hospital with our baby. Thankfully, my partner was able to be there as my one permitted support person. As we had done with our first labour, we played Yahtzee, we cuddled, but this time, we remembered our son.

If only all women were able to undergo the labour that I experienced. After the epidural was inserted at 5 cm, I merely felt pressure with contractions and could speak through them and even nap. After learning I was fully dilated, I had to slow down pushing because this baby was ready to enter the world. I pushed for only 10 minutes and once again, a beautiful baby landed on my chest, this time a girl. Zoe Dylan entered the world on a rainy day in March and a perfect rainbow arced over the hospital upon her arrival.

We will never get over the loss of our son, but it has taught us many things. Time is precious and so many things are out of our control, even our own bodies. Without the loss of our son, we wouldn't have our daughter right now. While that is an impossible truth to wrap our heads around, all we can do is be thankful for what we have, speak about him to our daughter, and smile that our rainbow came after the storm.

About Dana

Dana has been a registered nurse for 12 years and currently works at Kingston Health Sciences Centre. She lives in Kingston, Ontario with her partner Jay and together they have three children: Dylan, Zoe, and Gordon.

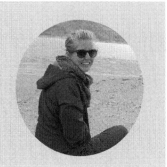

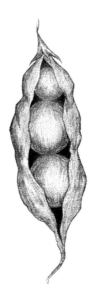

But will being too attentive to your newborn's cries make him manipulative? Fortunately, the answer to that question is "Hell no!"

—**Harvey Karp,** *The Happiest Baby on the Block: The New Way to Calm Crying and Help Your Newborn Baby Sleep Longer*

Reclaiming My Birth Story

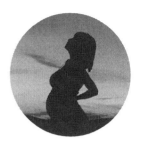

by Danielle BoByk
Kingston, Ontario

My daughter was opinionated from day one. After the anatomy ultrasound, we found out she was head up instead of head down – frank breech, to be specific. We were told not to worry, that she had plenty of time to turn around, but at the end of every appointment, my midwives would find her in the same spot: head up, bum down, feet to the right. By 30 weeks, I started researching ways to help her turn and implemented every technique I could. At 34 weeks, we scheduled an External Cephalic Version (ECV). At 37 weeks, two doctors tried and failed to manually turn my baby into the correct position. She would not budge. My midwives told me she just wanted to be up close to my chest so she could listen to my heartbeat; my husband and I joked that she had inherited his poor sense of direction.

Once the ECV failed, we were presented with two options; attempt a vaginal breech delivery or schedule a C-section. My midwives were positive about the outcome of a vaginal delivery, but the obstetric resident was less so. It quickly became clear to my husband and I that the staff at the hospital were not overly comfortable with that option, especially where I was a first-time mom. It seemed highly likely that I would end up with a caesarean regardless, only now with higher risks due to it being unplanned. So, we opted for the scheduled C-section and were booked in for two weeks later.

Making this choice was surprisingly emotional for me. I am pro-intervention when needed, and I had long since accepted the potential of a caesarean birth. But in all the times I had imagined how the birth of my baby would go, I had always pictured myself at least attempting a vaginal delivery. In fact, I had put a lot of effort into preparing for one. I had taken a prenatal class to learn strategies for managing pain, with the intent of attempting to go without an epidural. I had eaten six dates per day for the entirety of my third trimester because my midwife had said it might help make labour go faster. I had gone to yoga classes and on walks to keep my body in the best shape possible. Hearing my C-section described as "elective" was like a knife in my heart – I didn't want to have one, but it seemed to be the safest option for both me and my baby.

Over the next few days, I mourned the loss of the birth experience I thought I would have, as well as what I perceived to be the loss of my birth story. For years, I had watched my friends connect and bond over their stories of going into labour, giving birth, and everything that happened in between. None of my close friends or family had had a C-section, so there was no one who could relate to what I was going through. What kind of story would I have to tell when this was over? There was going to be no empowering tale of giving everything I had to bring my child into this world. I was simply going to go to the hospital, and they were going to take my baby out of me, with little involvement on my part.

The day arrived, and to some extent, my worries came true. On paper, my delivery was clinical. I showed up at the hospital on the allotted day at the allotted time and was prepped for surgery. I was given an epidural that numbed me from the waist down, leaving me able to feel pressure but not much else. My husband has a history of fainting at the sight of blood, so they put the curtain up high, and we chose to leave it up throughout the procedure – we did not want to risk having a second patient in the operating room. I did not see, or even really feel, my daughter being born.

However, that description does not do justice to how everyone in that room made sure to involve me in the birth of my child as much as possible. The anesthesiologist stayed standing throughout, watching over the curtain and letting me know when a hand made an appearance, and then a foot, and then the rest of our sweet little baby. The doctors immediately started describing her to my husband and I, telling us how alert she was and how big her eyes were. One of my midwives used my phone to take pictures so I could witness her birth after the fact. The other let us know where to look so she could show us our child before she was whisked off to be weighed and examined. The midwives placed my daughter on my chest for skin-to-skin as quickly as possible, and one of them stayed close to hold a protective hand over her so she did not get bumped by the surgeon's elbow.

When I tell my birth story, I do not simply say that I went to the hospital and they took a baby out of me. I talk about the whole medical team coming together to make a plan, just in case my husband passed out. I talk about my midwife holding my shoulders and coaching me all through the epidural procedure. I talk about the anesthesiologist giving me his fingers to hold on to when things got intense. I talk about the bizarre feeling of my baby's limbs and the surgeons' fingers moving around in my abdomen – like an octopus flailing all its tentacles simultaneously. I talk about how I started feeling pain towards the end, how the anesthesiologist eventually put me out for a few minutes using nitrous oxide, and what a weird trip that was.

When I tell my birth story, I share how incredibly alert my daughter was right from the start – something every single person commented on that first day of her life. I share how she tried to root the instant she was set on my chest. I share how she held onto her toes as she breastfed for the first time, still preferring to hang out in that frank breech position. I share how her legs would shoot up just about over her head when she was unswaddled.

When I tell my birth story, I explain how I navigated breastfeeding while still numb from the waist down and the incredible amount of positioning it took – pillows to hold me in place, rolled up blankets to hold my daughter in place, one hand supporting her and the other hand keeping my breast in the right spot. I explain how the wonderful nurses helped me with everything from breastfeeding to using the bathroom. I explain how my amazing husband supported me throughout the surgery and took over almost all of the baby care in the early days of my recovery.

When I tell my birth story, I relive the incredible and unique experience of bringing my daughter into this world.

In the end, I view my decision to have a caesarean birth as one of my first true acts as a mother: letting go of what I wanted in favour of what was best for my child. But when it comes down to it, I had mourned the loss of something that I will never truly miss. I may not be able to bond with friends over whether or not our waters broke and what labour was like, but I can bond with them over the feeling of finally getting to meet our babies and the struggle of adjusting to life with a newborn. I carried my daughter within me for nine months, and I underwent major surgery to birth her as safely as possible. I was so fortunate to be surrounded by people who went above and beyond to make that experience the best it could possibly be.

I may not have a traditional birth story, but that doesn't mean I don't have one at all. I still have a story to tell, and it's one that I'm proud to share.

About Danielle

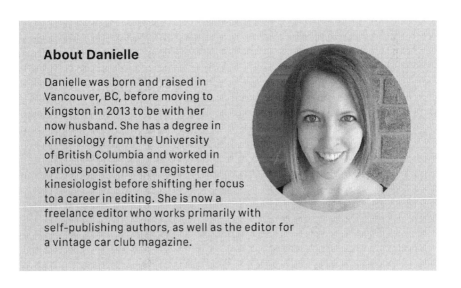

Danielle was born and raised in Vancouver, BC, before moving to Kingston in 2013 to be with her now husband. She has a degree in Kinesiology from the University of British Columbia and worked in various positions as a registered kinesiologist before shifting her focus to a career in editing. She is now a freelance editor who works primarily with self-publishing authors, as well as the editor for a vintage car club magazine.

Believing in Your Body

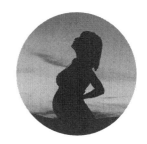

by Jenna Kovacic
Richmond Hill, Ontario

When my son was born, a part of me was born too.

My journey started in March of 2016, when my husband and I found out we were expecting. I was scared, but not because it was finally happening but because something didn't feel right. I was feeling off, almost like it wasn't real, and I kept looking at my positive test, trying to convince myself that it was. I had the strangest feeling that I would be pregnant again in a few months with a boy, but I didn't understand why I felt that way; I was pregnant now.

At seven weeks, we found out it was an ectopic pregnancy. I was never meant to have this baby, and that's why I never truly felt pregnant or connected. I was devastated. I had wanted to be a mother for as long as I could remember. I allowed myself to grieve and then I really started to care for myself, emotionally and physically.

Two months later, I was pregnant with a little boy, just like I felt I would be. The time had come to change my thought patterns and face the fear of the unknown. I was ready to go deep and prepare myself for what I knew would be a challenging but exciting experience.

At my first midwife appointment, she seemed to be looking forever for his heartbeat, and then she finally said, "Ah, your hearts are beating together," and then I got it. We would have to work together, always.

I was eager the entire pregnancy for the birth; it was all I could think about. I dreamed of a successful home birth and devoured every book on the subject. I used hypnobirthing and kept visualizing how it could go. At 40 weeks and 6 days, I went into labour. My husband put a plate of dinner in front of me and my first real contraction hit. I remember laughing and saying, "Whoa, if this gets any worse, I may not be able to handle it!" My body and mind were going to test me in ways it never had before, just a few hours from then.

I called my midwives and they told me to take a nap and relax. I couldn't do any of those things, so I took a shower, shaved my legs, and put some comfy clothes on. I hydrated as much as I could and tried to eat, but I was experiencing incredible back labour. The midwives arrived around midnight, excited to see me eating and in good spirits. Shortly after, I was in active labour and having intense, strong contractions.

As the contractions became more intense, I was transported into the "labour world." I was somewhere else and became someone else. I wasn't nervous at all like I thought I would be, I had all the confidence in the world that my body would do what it was supposed to. I laboured in the shower, on the bed with some music, in the bathroom, and on a birthing stool. I was on this magical ride, feeling every wave, and I kept saying yes to it all. My body felt powerful and strong. I let myself go, allowing my body to do the work it needed to bring my baby to me. I vividly remember falling asleep between contractions, which could have only been a few minutes, yet I felt like I had slept for an hour.

After 15 hours, it was time to push, and we were so excited! My midwife told me our baby would be with us soon. So, I started pushing, and pushing, and pushing, and nothing was happening. I saw the midwives look at each other because they didn't understand why it was taking so long. I would push with each contraction and I slowly, but surely, started to wear myself out. I had two midwives and they ended up calling two more for support. I tried different positions, and nothing helped, but not once did I waver. I knew I could do it. I just needed more time.

A few more hours of pushing and they saw his head wasn't completely turned; he was coming out on the side. I lay in bed, my husband next to me, sweating, a cold cloth on my forehead while the midwives fed me fruit and tea for hydration and energy. I kept pushing with everything I had, every ounce of energy, every muscle in my body. I didn't know pushing could be so hard. At one point, all four midwives were standing, kneeling, and sitting next to me while my husband paced the room, all coming up with different ideas on things we could try. After each contraction, and another push that didn't bring me my baby, I collapsed on the bed, unsure of how long I had been pushing. The room was still, and I could feel the energy pulsing. Everyone's eyes were on me. Was I going to do it? Could I do it? What would happen? My midwife said, "Look, the sun is coming up." I had no idea it was already the next day.

My husband suggested the hospital numerous times, but I knew my baby was okay and I so badly wanted to have him at home. His heart rate was steady and strong, and he was cool as a cucumber, still wiggling around like he always had, waiting to meet us. I had been telling my son days before that I was going to be brave for him and I wasn't going to let him or myself down. Things started to slow, and my contractions were further apart, but the support and positivity in that room never changed. My husband sat behind me, cradling me, whispering, "Come on, you can do this" over and over. His sweet tone kept reminding me to be relaxed and stay in this. Everyone in that room encouraged me to keep going, to not give up, and to find the strength wherever I could.

I'll never forget the moment everything shifted. I was sweating, exhausted, and sitting on a birthing stool, which wasn't helping. My doula grabbed my hand, looked me in the eyes, and said with firmness and so much warmth, "You can do this. Let's do this." I got back on the bed, and I pushed but this time, the pushing felt different. I pushed from what felt like the depths of my soul. Everything I had left went into those pushes. Unlike before, when I had been quiet during my pushing, I let out a roar like no other. I didn't realize how much I had been holding back. That strong push was what we needed, and it moved his head out! I gave another big push and felt the rest of him slide out of my body. I heard a midwife say, "12:57." Just as I looked up, they were placing my big, beautiful, pink, sweet boy on my chest. My husband's eyes filled with tears, and everyone looked so relieved.

Forty-one weeks of growing this little soul in my body, nourishing him, loving him, keeping him safe, and then finally bringing him into the world. I've been attached to him from the moment we made him. I am forever grateful for the most raw, emotional, and empowering experience of my life. My son's birth story is a true testament to what your mind and body can overcome, along with the right support system. I knew right after I gave birth to him that I wanted to experience this again, and I did, in July 2019. We welcomed a beautiful baby girl in our home, in the same bed her brother was born in, with the same support and care.

To my son and daughter, I know we were waiting for each other and I'm so glad we are finally all together.

About Jenna

Jenna is enjoying life with her husband, son, and daughter. After her first birth experience, she knew she needed to do something with her newfound passion and so, she became a doula. She is a promoter of self-care, a lover of meditation, simple living, books, any outdoor activity, and tries to be as present as possible in her everyday life. You can reach her on Facebook or Instagram: @over.the.moon.birth

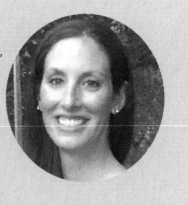

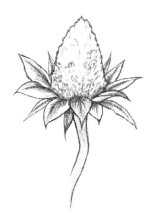

The best way I know to counter the effects of frightening stories is to hear or read empowering ones. I mean stories that change you because you read or heard them, because the teller of the story taught you something you didn't know before or helped you look at things from a different angle than you ever had before ... Stories teach us in ways we can remember.

—Ina May Gaskin,
Ina May's Guide to Childbirth

Mother Knows Best

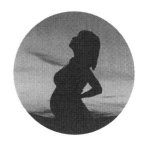

by Julie Meier
Calgary, Alberta

As I waddled out of the exam room, I happened to look over at the white board above the nurses' station. There, written in black marker, was the following: "Room 4 - Labour?"

That was me.

Was I in labour? Yes.

No question mark needed.

This was my third child and, though every birth is different, I came in with a certain amount of knowledge and expectation. That night, by the time my husband, Dan, had finished watching a play-off hockey game and I had spent a few hours sleeping fitfully, I knew I was in labour.

We called our friend, Kelly, to come and spend the night with our other two children, who were already tucked in bed, and off we went.

As we arrived at the hospital, with the digital green glow of our truck's dash announcing the ungodly hour of 2 a.m., we were directed to labour and delivery for an assessment.

"I think you've got a while to go," the nurse stated from her position between my legs. "Why don't you just go home and get some rest until things have progressed further?"

There are times in your life when you need to dismiss expectations—your own and others—and listen to your gut. Mine was telling me that, although I may not have measured above 4 cm dilated at that point, my baby's arrival was imminent.

"No, I think we are here to stay," I said, knowing full well that we would get home to the farm with barely enough time to turn around and return to this exact spot. So, we settled into Room 4 and prepared to wait it out.

Time wavered for a while, as it tends to do when you are caught in that strange land between pain and excitement. Possibly an hour and a half passed – just long enough to have driven to our farm and then raced back into the city again.

By then, the contractions were becoming more insistent, and I suggested it was high time for my husband to go and find a nurse for a reassessment. That set into motion a series of events, which included a shocked assessment nurse, a hastily procured wheelchair, and a quick glimpse at that blasted question mark.

It was still there, leering at me, as they wheeled me out of Room 4, through the reception area and down the hall to the birthing rooms. We passed mothers-to-be who were just arriving, clearly in the early stage of labour, still looking cool as cucumbers. I, however, was feeling slightly less than cool at that point as I gripped the arms of the wheelchair tightly and another contraction took hold.

My husband was sent to properly admit me (they really didn't believe I was in labour, did they?) and in doing so, nearly missed the birth. A nurse suggested I step into the warm shower to relax my muscles and help progress labour, and progress it did. The nurse stepped away for a few minutes and, when she returned, I was met with another look of surprise.

"Why are you pushing?" she asked.

Clearly, April 28 was the day for questions.

But Katelyn was not interested in waiting for questions to be answered, and neither was I. Just after 4 a.m., she made her debut in the world—bloody and beautiful, messy and perfect—my little redheaded girl. Suddenly, the questions didn't matter anymore because my wait was over, and all the answers I needed lay cradled in my arms.

Fourteen years have passed since that day, and any memory of the pain has faded until it is nothing but a faint shadow but the joy has remained just as palpable as the day I first met her. That question mark on the whiteboard? I still think about it occasionally.

I have learned many lessons as a mother, but one of the most important is knowing the power of instinct. It is easy to get caught up in worry and doubt, and to give in to the thoughts and opinions of others, but motherly instinct trumps all. As a shy and reserved person, I have often struggled to speak up, but have learned to advocate for myself and my children when needed and to let my instincts guide my decisions.

We, as mothers, are inherently strong and intuitive. We really do know best.

About Julie

Julie was born and raised in Calgary, and now lives on a farm where she can enjoy a view of the Calgary skyline and Rocky Mountains as she writes at her kitchen table. Her work has been published in several online journals and she has been shortlisted for a number of flash fiction story contests. When she is not writing, you might find Julie outside cuddling sheep, or devising new ways to embarrass her teenagers. You can follow Julie at Twitter @Julie_M_Meier.

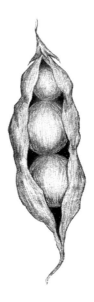

Other people in her community would feed her, nurture her, and take all responsibilities off her plate so that she could focus on one thing only; transitioning healthily and happily from expectant woman to mother.

— **Heng Ou,** *The First 40 Days*

A Full Moon Eclipse Birth

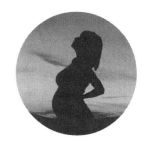

by Kristin Nuttall
Pemberton, British Columbia

My darling angel baby, I want to tell you about your birth.

They say that when the student is ready, the teacher appears. This student spent years trying to conceive you by wishing, praying, inviting, dreaming, and manifesting. From lifestyle changes like modifying diet, taking herbs, and receiving acupuncture, to the well-known local secret of eating lots and lots of Pemberton potatoes (which, by the way, could be the reason that Pemberton has the second-highest birth rate next to Idaho. Interestingly, they get their seed potatoes from Pemberton). Finally, inverting my body seemed to be what worked, or maybe it was the combination of everything? I remember the time of your conception, when your glamma (on Daddy's side) unknowingly entered into the room without knocking during our vacation to the Island. Little did she realize why I was upside down and barely covered.

Your daddy knew of your presence before I did, when, a couple of weeks later, I thought I had food poisoning from our sushi date. Our Chinese medicine doctor, the infamous Sunny Lee, said from the pulses that you were a boy or possibly a strong-willed female. Leading up to the birth process, I did every movement possible with the "Spinning Babies" exercises to get you into optimal positioning. Meanwhile, you had already been there, waiting in position for many months. I learned in my schooling of biodynamic craniosacral and perinatal psychology training about a baby's clockwise rotation descending through the mother's pelvic stations; that, if started from a left side lay, it would be easier to find the optimal occiput-anterior birthing positioning. I wanted to protect your safe passage by doing everything I could to avoid any medical interventions. I wanted to create space for you to smoothly negotiate past the tight soft tissue and bones. I visualized you being there with your head tucked, chin in, and your arms crossed over your chest. We co-created your beautiful birth. We did it together! I am completely in awe of you and will always be.

At long last, the estimated date of your arrival had come, and a few days had gone by. I was feeling ready, but we hadn't quite finished preparing everything. You waited until all details were in place. Your support team was assembled, the car was packed, the freezer was stocked, my belly-cast was done, and your nursery and co-sleeper bassinet were all ready for you. We decided to make our way to Squamish to my dear friend's home. She had had three home births and she offered to vacate the house with her family to go stay with her new man. It was an offer we couldn't refuse. Your glamma and auntie (on my side) were busy cooking and cleaning for three more days. We had time to set up all that we might have possibly needed, even down to the sterilized towels sealed in brown paper bags. I was taking evening primrose oil and having your daddy doing perineal stretching with birthing oil. In lieu of sitting on a tractor, I bounced on the trampoline (which I got in trouble for). I drank tea and needled my thumbs all in hopes of bringing on your birth. I think the acupuncture could have helped. Then again, you knew exactly the moment you were waiting for was when the full moon rose on our horizon as a visible eclipse.

There was some bright red spotting, it was just after 5 p.m. on July 15th, 2019. I excitedly hopped in the bath and slowly felt the sensations coming on. I ate a huge meal to give me energy for the marathon ahead. I got in the shower again. I stared out the window at the beautiful moon. I had patience and we waited for your arrival. Our whole family had completely taken over my friend's house. I crawled into her bed with a shower curtain placed thoughtfully under the sheets to protect the mattress. Your daddy was still at our house with the doggies in Pemberton. At about 1 a.m., I called him and said, "This is happening soon. Please bring my red dolphin-wolf to comfort me." Until he arrived, it was so special to spend time with glamma; she felt honoured to be there with me. In the spirit of honesty without wanting to offend, I had let her know in advance that if I felt her anxiety around this home birth scenario or any incongruence, that I might ask her or anyone else in the room to leave. It was comforting to know that she understood. I learned that the wonderful thing about supporting a birthing woman is that no one should take any offence to anything.

Resting between surges through the night, I gathered strength and curled up by my mom; your daddy arrived at about 3 a.m. Things got intense around 5 a.m. and I needed your daddy's continuous pressure on my hip flexors for every cresting wave of contraction. By 7:30 a.m., I called our doula who was also a 3rd-year midwifery student at UBC. She arrived by 9 a.m., filled the pool, and I hopped in. It really was an "aquadural," as they say. Your glamma tuned into the ancient ritual of continuously boiling water for the birth pool. Your auntie kept bringing the warm water to add in to keep me warm. There was music, candles, and a whole table of comfort resources, but I forgot about them all. The only thing that mattered was that pressure on my hip flexors, which had then been taken over by my doula. Your amazing dad moved from his three-hour post at my hips to support my quivering jaw so he could reassure me and coach me. I was so proud of him that he knew instinctively to do that. I declined checking dilation in advance. I knew it would only make me anxious and take me out of the body-entrusted state I was in. Around 10 a.m., about 15 hours into it, something had changed. I felt what must have been "cranial moulding." My pelvic floor bulged like a hammock, then retracted, and I wasn't doing a thing. I thought it was time to call the midwife.

She arrived in 20 minutes and had to inform me there was no OB that could do an emergency C-section in Squamish and now was our last chance to drive to Vancouver (just in case). I said, "Thanks, I'm good here." I went back to your birth song – making the sounds of my deep, primal brain, where I had complete trust in my body and in you, my baby. I felt a wooden tool in the water against my belly to listen to your heart tones. This made me happy. I didn't ever want to use a doppler.

One thing that kept ringing in my mind was not to push at all until my body did so naturally. I see how that can help keep the perineum intact, which was true for me. Your daddy held my jaw, telling me I was beautiful and kissing me. I told him to kiss me with some tongue. He remembers me yelling that boldly at him and he was a little embarrassed in front of the family. The hormones of his kiss took me into a respite of joy and peace. I kept looking at my beautiful wolfie pup lying beside me, being relaxed, and I could relax a little more too.

Your head crowned and popped right out. I let out one surprise shriek as my left labia tore superficially for a split second that was barely painful. Lucky for me, I think the "ring of fire" feeling that some women get was completely offset by the water. Then, it was truly a moment suspended in time. I had my hand on your head and the midwife brought her hand there too. I thought she was turning your head, so I swatted her hand away, telling her not to touch, but it was *you* corkscrewing your shoulders out. On the next wave of my fascinating expulsion reflexes, my doula cued me, saying you were about to come into my arms and that I could push during the next contraction. I said, "Really?" So, I directed my breath, bearing down. I felt total relief as you came out and the midwife said, "Catch baby, catch baby…"

Then, I brought you onto my chest and you didn't even cry. We gazed into each other's eyes with full clarity, no drops to blur your vision in seeing me. Your colour and reflexes were good; still not a peep. It was the undisturbed golden hour. I couldn't take my eyes off your eyes. It felt like the most important first face-to-face imprinting chat. Your daddy said, "holy smokes" over and over. He checked and announced that you were a girl. He named you Winnie. Warm towels were draped over us, and I encouraged you to do the breast-crawl, moving up my belly. You bobbed your head around and you found the big bull's eye, unassisted for your first feed. It was total bliss. About 30-45 minutes later, our midwife said the cord had pulsed out. She felt the slack of the cord and tightening of my uterus. She gently guided the placenta down and it followed out without my noticing further contractions. I chose not to stitch the tiny superficial tear, as it would have only been for esthetic purposes.

Your glamma prepared the bedroom with fresh sheets, flowers, candles, and delicious, nibbly food. Your daddy took off his shirt and held you while I rinsed off in the shower. We all crawled into the bed with a platter of treats.

I continued to enjoy the firsts of you, my darling, as you fed and slept on my glowing heartbeat with peace and quiet. Your glamma and auntie made sure I stayed in bed, and they hurried about cooking and cleaning.

My dear friend, whose home we were in, had arrived moments after you were born while we were still in the birthing pool. She quietly supported and went to work dehydrating and encapsulating your placenta.

Gentle fawn, meeting you was the most beautiful day of my life. We celebrated you with a fancy birthing-day cake as you nuzzled skin-to-skin inside my shirt. We stayed there in Squamish for another week, resting and being together in the splendour of newborn moments.

We are so blessed by all the support and care we had. My doula and the midwives visited us at the house every day for seven days. They all said you had "a beautiful and gentle birth." Your auntie, being a postpartum doula, prepared a daily herbal sitz bath with comfrey root. She wrapped my belly in long cotton fabric to aid in reshaping my torso, she put cool cabbage leaves on my breasts as my milk came in, and cooked nourishing foods based on the 4th-trimester traditions to assist in milk-making.

They stayed by our side for six weeks with a camper parked in the front yard of our house. Your grandmother was right when she said that with your birth, I would experience a deeper level of love than I had ever known. Your daddy and I love you more than we could have ever imagined. Thank you for choosing us. This story, dear Winnie, is a gift to you for your first birthday.

Love,

Mom

About Kristin

Kristin has had the opportunity to attend many births as a doula and biodynamic craniosacral therapist. The more she learned about birth, the greater her reverence became and the greater her passion grew in assisting mothers to have empowered birthing experiences. Kristin's greatest birthing support mentor is Gloria Lemay from Vancouver BC. Many women of the Sea-to-Sky corridor had birthed "Gloria babies." Kristin took the "Wise Woman Way of Birth" and "Birth Takes a Village."

Through the Doula's Eyes: A Photo Story

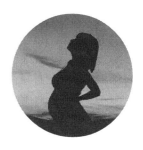

by Jessica Cheyne
Woodstock, Ontario

This birth was not only my first one to support, but it was also my first one to capture.

Forty-one weeks to the day, and Mom was eager to meet her first daughter. She had three boys waiting at home and a husband who was also anxiously waiting for their daughter's arrival.

This client was also a good friend of mine; a headstrong, exhausted woman just waiting for the pregnancy to be over. I kept saying to her, "You are one of the strongest women I know. So, what do you think your daughter is going to be like?" She was politely impatient—as most pregnant people are—and I can't blame her, I know that feeling from my own pregnancies.

I picked her up at 7:45 a.m. on February 15th, 2020, and we headed to the hospital. She was set to be induced at 8:00 a.m. The morning was cold and stiff, but the excitement in her eyes melted it all away. When we arrived at the hospital, I grabbed our bags and walked through the wind into the front doors; this is when I started to doubt my abilities. *Am I going to be what she needs? Is she going to regret not having her husband here? Do I know enough?*

She got herself checked in and we walked into the labour and delivery room, putting all our stuff on the floor like we were just staying at a hotel for the night. This part of the hospital had a relaxing atmosphere, and it was quiet, as she was the only one giving birth that day.

Her doctor came in and broke her water right away. She was only 2 cm at this point, and I thought to myself, *the baby will be here today!* Contractions started pretty fast; they were irregular, but they were there. She decided to relax in the tub before they got more intense. I believe she wanted one last moment to feel as one. We went through a few positions to help with the contractions, and she was breathing well through them.

The plan was to go as natural as possible. She had had three epidurals with her other children, so she really wanted to try without one, and that she did. But there came a time when she knew that if she didn't get an epidural sooner than later, she would not be in the right headspace for when her baby was born, and that was the last thing she wanted, for both of them.

I supported her mentally and physically as the anesthesiologist started the process. This was the best decision for her and that's all that mattered. Once the epidural was set in place, she got comfortable in her bed, and within two hours, she was at 9 cm. That excitement turned to discouragement when it took another four hours to be ready to push.

The baby's position was right occiput transverse (ROT) and the nurse was unaware. We didn't find out until the head nurse came in and performed her own check. Once the nurse knew why the baby wasn't moving into position, she called the doctor who then performed another cervical exam.

"You're going to have your baby now," said the head nurse. With the next contraction, she was told to push, and the doctor guided the baby into the right position, which got her to 10 cm quickly.

At this point, she was completely over with the day and everything that had transpired over the last 10 hours. Tired, exhausted, anxious, excited, and 100% emotional. She needed a moment to gather herself. Once she took that final deep breath in, she gave it all she had. Within four to five pushes, her daughter entered the world.

THROUGH THE DOULA'S EYES: A PHOTO STORY

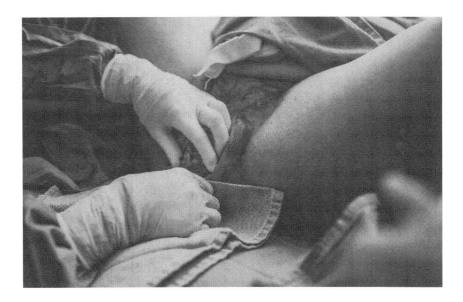

My first birth as a doula is going to stay with me forever. I witnessed a friend and a mom welcome her fourth healthy child, a daughter she always wanted, into her arms. The day was filled with laughter, love, and learning experiences, and I will always be grateful to have had the honour of being present at the beautiful birth of Baby F.

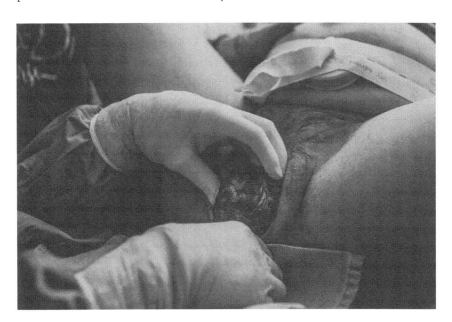

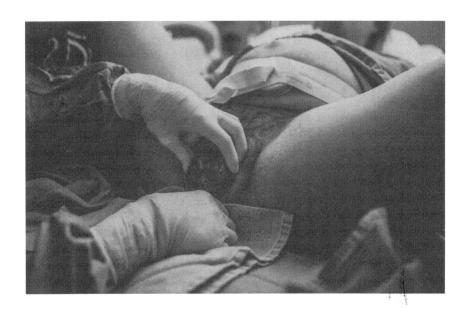
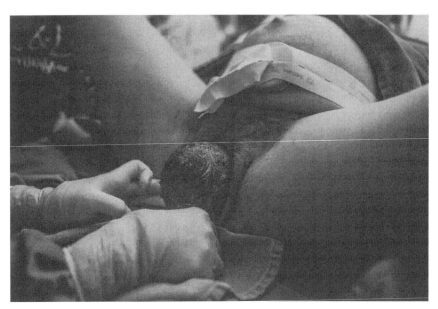

THROUGH THE DOULA'S EYES: A PHOTO STORY

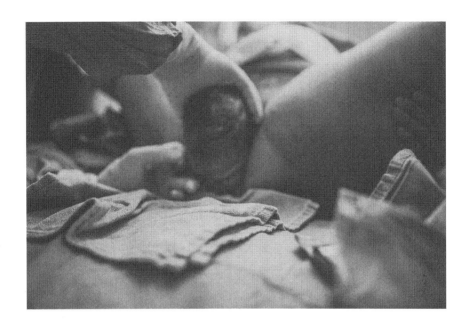

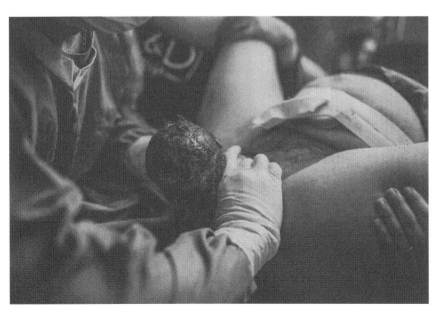

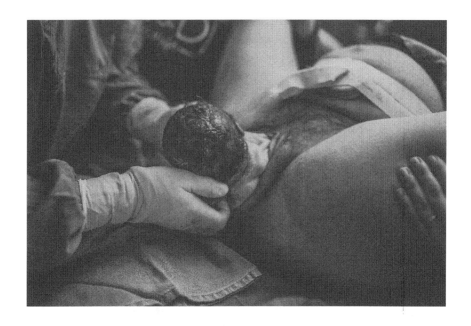

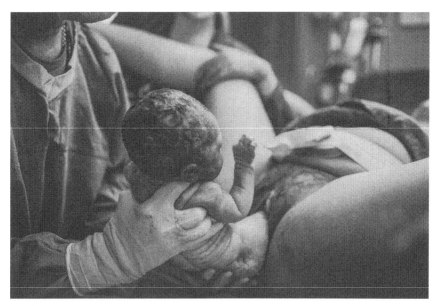

THROUGH THE DOULA'S EYES: A PHOTO STORY

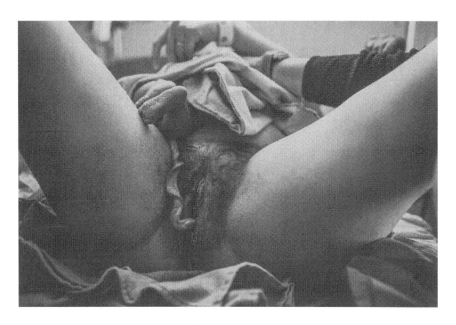

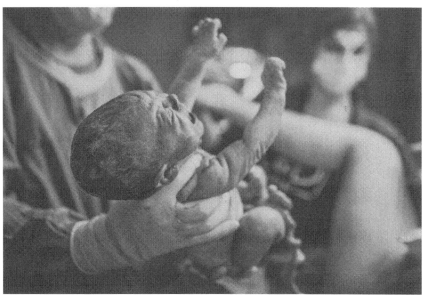

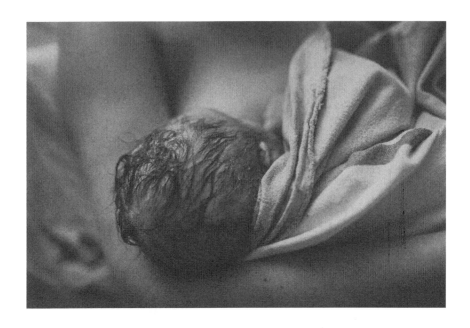

About Jessica

Jessica is the owner of Soothe Doula Services. What motivated her to start it was hearing the stories of many birthing people and their journeys, many of them negative and trying. She knew there was a way to help curve the fear that came along with labour and delivery. Having three difficult labours and births herself, she felt it was time to educate not only herself, but also others on how to have a birth that they would be happy to share and remember. Jessica lives in Woodstock, Ontario. She is also the owner of Jarful Refillery. You can follow her @jarfulrefillery.

Just Like Hollywood

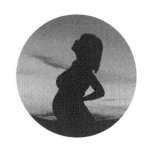

by Alison Ryder
Kingston, Ontario

"Remember, babies are born on their birth date, not their due date! And it doesn't happen like it does in Hollywood!" These were the parting words of wisdom I took home with me as we left our two-day intensive weekend childbirth class.

At that time, I was 34 weeks and 5 days, so when my water broke while making dinner, I recognized the signs—it was just a few hours since the class—but I was also quite skeptical.

It started as a trickle, and I wasn't sure if it was just extra vaginal discharge. I went to the bathroom to tidy up, but right after I thought the leaking had stopped, it started again. I decided to make a dash for the bedroom, where I could change my underwear and put on a pad. A big one.

My partner was in the kitchen. "Honey, can you come with me, please? Now," I said as I passed him. I didn't wait for a reply and don't even think I looked at him. (He thought he was in trouble for something, and later told me that he immediately went through everything he'd done recently to try to figure out what I was mad about.)

He followed me to the bedroom. "I think my water broke?" I said, still not quite believing what was happening. I hadn't had any contractions, nor had there been any sign that things weren't progressing normally. The baby wasn't due for another five weeks, and I had been sure she would be late. In my family, babies are always late.

"Do you want me to call the midwife?" he asked, concerned.

"No, I think we should- Can you get me a towel?" I replied as I felt a fresh gush of fluid between my legs.

He dashed to the bathroom and grabbed one, which I promptly sat on. "Yeah, I think maybe we should call the midwife!"

The midwife said she would meet us at the clinic, not far from our house, to test to see if it was amniotic fluid.

It was, as it turned out, amniotic fluid.

We drove over to the local hospital, only a few minutes away. On the way there, I thought I started to feel what were probably contractions; they felt like mild menstrual cramps at the time. We went into the non-emergency entrance of the hospital and walked into the labour and delivery wing. Because I wasn't in active labour yet, they had me sit in the triage area where they monitor the women in early labour.

A doctor came to visit and explained that they wanted the baby out within 48 hours because the amniotic sac had ruptured. However, they didn't want the baby out too soon because the baby's lungs were probably underdeveloped. They hooked me up to an IV and gave me some antibiotics in addition to some steroids that they hoped would give the baby a little boost before she came out.

At this point, the doctor did not actually check my cervix. They wanted the baby to stay in as long as possible, so they didn't want to introduce any potential infections or irritants. Besides, my contractions were still mild.

The doctor and the nurses were not in any kind of hurry. We all expected that I would be there for a day or two, so my midwife went home to try to get some sleep before the next day's labour.

My partner took this opportunity to check in with some friends. In our haste to leave, we didn't have everything we needed, nor had we eaten dinner, and had friends stop by the house, pick a few things up, and grab some fast food for us. The nurses said I should probably eat if I felt hungry because I was going to be in for a long night.

Our friends arrived around 8:30 p.m. and stuck around for a while (still in the triage area) while we ate. My contractions were starting to ramp up a little, enough for me to be able to identify when they started and when they ended, so I started timing them.

After a while, I started to feel nauseous and vomited everything I just ate. The nurse thought it was a side-effect of some of the drugs they gave me and gave me some anti-nausea medication in my IV drip. My contractions were also ramping up. My partner asked if I wanted to play cards and I said sure, but by the time he had found them in the bag and started shuffling, I had changed my mind. Cards didn't sound fun anymore.

By 10:00 p.m., the contractions were quite strong. I was starting to panic a little – how bad were these contractions going to get? I didn't really want to get an epidural (I'm terrified of needles), but if I was going to be here for a long time and the contractions were just going to keep building and building, I was definitely going to need some pain relief sometime soon.

I had been timing my contractions at 3.5 minutes apart, lasting about 45 seconds. The nurse called the doctor back and checked my cervix for the first time. My partner was expecting the worst, and predicted that I was only 3 cm dilated, while I was more optimistically hoping for 6 cm. We were both shocked—as were the doctor and nurse—when he exclaimed, "Wow, you're fully dilated!"

That's when everyone sprang into action. I was having a baby right now. The nurses helped me to a wheelchair and told me, in no uncertain terms, not to push yet. They had to get me to a delivery room first.

I was transferred to the delivery bed and the room was already full of medical staff, including a team from the Neonatal Intensive Care Unit (NICU), ready to collect a premature baby. Someone called my midwife but warned me that she might not be back in time for the delivery, so an obstetrician was going to step in and take care of things.

If I'd really thought about it, I might have been upset that my midwife wasn't there, but to be honest, I hadn't really been mentally prepared for labour yet. I didn't really have a plan or expectations of what I wanted my labour to be like, or who I wanted to be there. My partner and I hadn't practiced what his role was going to be. In the moment, though, everything was happening so quickly. My partner was there, my friends were still in the waiting room, and I was surrounded by a team that was going to make sure my baby and I were healthy and safe. That was the most important thing.

Then, I was told I should start pushing, and everyone waited expectantly, sure that the baby was going to pop right out in record time.

Turns out, that was not to be the case.

I started pushing, still completely unmedicated, but quickly asked what was still available for pain management. I didn't realize that the pain from contractions would feel different than the pain from pushing a baby through the birth canal, though I can't say I'm a fan of either. I had originally hoped for a tub (our local hospital has delivery rooms for water birthing) but with a premature baby, that option was off the table. An epidural was right out, since things were happening way too fast. So, I was given nitrous oxide, which was really the only option I had available.

It took me a while to get the hang of pushing. I had trouble with pushing and breathing and counting to the 5 or 10 seconds that the nurses were asking me to push for. (I'll be honest, the laughing gas wasn't helping me focus.)

My partner was right next to me the whole time. One time, he made a joke about leaving to go to the bathroom, and I just stared at him, wondering why he would say such a thing at a time like this. Turns out, laughing gas does not make you think everything is funny. Mostly, though, he held my hand while I squeezed it in a death grip—there may have been bruising—and said pleasant things to me. I wasn't really listening. At one point, I told him, "Honey, I have no idea what you're saying, but I like hearing your voice, so keep talking to me."

At first, I was making good progress, but then I started to stall. I'd push and the baby would descend the birth canal, but in between pushes, she would recede inside. The team was monitoring the baby, of course, and eventually, the obstetrician told me that the baby was now in distress, and he wanted to perform an episiotomy.

I have a great fear of surgery and medical procedures in general, so when I had learned about episiotomies in the childbirth class, I had immediately turned to my partner and said, "Let's try to avoid that, please!"

So, when the doctor suggested it, even though I was a little loopy from the drugs, even though I was in pain, tired, wanted the baby out, and was not doing a great job at pushing, I said, loudly, "No, I do not want that."

To the doctor's credit, he immediately said, "Okay, then." And just like that, they weren't going to do an episiotomy, because I didn't want one. Then, he added, "But that means you're going to have to push harder."

Apparently, that was all the motivation I needed, and my daughter was born less than 10 minutes later. It wasn't even midnight yet.

So, although she was right about other things, the doula from our childbirth class was wrong on one count. Births can and do happen like in Hollywood – water breaks at home, rush to the hospital, a little bit of pushing while friends anxiously sit around in the waiting room, and then, like magic, a baby appears!

About Aly

Aly Ryder is a Canadian advisor on policies and programs that help the homeless. She's lived in Kingston, Ontario for 16 years, since attending Queen's University. In her spare time, she enjoys hiking, ultimate frisbee, and board games. This is her fifth pregnancy and first birth.

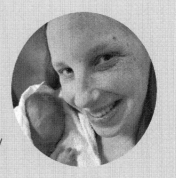

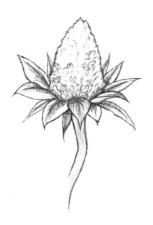

Research shows that women vividly recall their birth experiences for many years ... None has complete control over pregnancy and childbirth, but the decisions you make during pregnancy will affect your memory of your birth experience.

   —**Penny Simkin,** *Pregnancy, Childbirth and the Newborn – The Complete Guide*

A Dramatic Debut

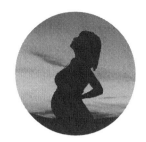

by Sara Wettlaufer
Hamilton/Brantford, Ontario

On Friday, March 8th, 2019, I was looking forward to my last day of work before starting maternity leave. The day went by without incident, and I was determined to have a productive evening. My husband was away for work for the weekend so I figured that I would use my time alone to make a dent in the growing to-do list I hoped to complete before the baby was born. My due date was 15 days away and I figured there was plenty of time to get everything done. That night, I took my dogs for a walk, ate supper, cleaned the basement, and baked brownies. I also ate half of the pan of said brownies while watching television. Satisfied with my evening, I went to bed and fell asleep around 11:30 p.m.

I awoke abruptly around 1:00 a.m. to use the bathroom. Upon returning to bed, I noticed my stomach was feeling quite crampy. Of course, I had eaten all of those brownies, so I didn't think much of it. After a few minutes of discomfort, I realized that my "cramps" were coming and going in small waves. I sat up and began counting what were now certainly contractions.

I tracked my contractions for about 45 minutes before deciding to call my midwife. The contractions didn't seem to be spacing out, nor were they getting weaker. When one contraction literally brought me to my knees, I knew I needed to call. Once my midwife was on her way, I drew myself a bath and proceeded to call my parents and my in-laws, who left almost immediately, and then my husband. He and I decided to wait until my midwife assessed me before he left to come home. We figured it would be a long while before the baby arrived.

In the bathtub, the contractions were getting much stronger and I had mostly ditched my deep breathing techniques in favour of moaning and yelling. Since I had only been in labour for about an hour, I figured I was only a few centimetres dilated. If this was what early labour felt like, I really wasn't sure I would be able to handle much more.

My midwife arrived around 2:15 a.m. and helped me out of the tub to perform a cervical check. To my amazement, I was already 9 cm dilated. No wonder those last few contractions were so terrible! What I had thought was early labour was actually transition and I would be pushing shortly. My husband obviously needed to leave for home, but he would almost certainly miss the birth. My midwife also acknowledged that while I had wanted to have a hospital birth, she was worried we wouldn't make it in time and thought it was best to deliver the baby at home. The moment the words "9 cm" came out of her mouth, I knew the hospital birth plan was out the window. I was more than happy to oblige at her suggestion.

My parents arrived shortly after my midwife and my mom came upstairs to assist her in preparing our bedroom for a home birth. They then helped me out of the tub and onto the bed. I laboured on my hands and knees for a short while, until moving onto my side and eventually onto my back, propped up by pillows into a somewhat seated position. The backup midwife, who looks after the baby following birth, entered the scene. My husband's parents had arrived now as well, and my mother-in-law climbed onto the bed to help. The dads remained downstairs to preoccupy the dogs, who were getting rather curious about all of the commotion.

At this point, I was ready to push. My mom had put my husband on video chat with us as he drove home. His mother and the baby's midwife were holding my legs up while my midwife was in the middle, coaching me through. Everyone around me was fantastic about staying positive and encouraging me through each contraction and push. While there was still plenty of pain, being able to channel my energy into pushing felt far more productive than just breathing through contractions. Soon, the baby had reached a point where I would only need to push a couple more times to get the baby out. On the next push, I distinctly felt and saw the baby's head emerge. That gave me the motivation I needed and on the next contraction, I pushed the rest of the baby's body out. I had pushed for 40 minutes and my total time in labour was a mere three hours.

Immediate relief overwhelmed me as the baby was brought to my chest. The baby let out a small cry but settled as soon as they were laid on me. They were covered in fluid and blood, but it didn't matter, and I just stared in wonder and amazement. Of course, we still didn't know if the baby was a boy or a girl. My midwife tried to get the camera pointed for my husband to make the reveal, and in all the commotion, he made a quick guess. "Is it a girl?" My midwife confirmed his guess, and everyone erupted in excitement. We had just had our baby and it was a girl!

My mom cut the cord and my midwife began working to help me get the placenta out. They hooked me up with oxytocin to get the process started, but it didn't seem to be working. After a half-hour, paramedics were called to bring me to the hospital so I could deliver the placenta there. My husband arrived just as the paramedics did and raced upstairs to see us. Our little family had a couple of moments together, and then my husband was prompted to take over skin-to-skin as I was brought to the hospital.

As much as I was disappointed to have to leave my baby so soon, I knew she would be in good hands with her father. The baby was completely healthy, and I recognized that it was important for me to be healthy now so I could be there for her later. At the hospital, I was given more oxytocin but to no avail. The on-call obstetrician prepared me for a manual extraction while an operating room would be ready for a surgical removal, if needed. Neither option sounded appealing to me. As the doctor prepped the OR, my midwife had me push one more time. To all our relief, it worked, and the placenta was out.

Soon, my husband and the baby arrived. She had scored well on all her tests, so she was merely a visitor at the hospital and didn't have to be admitted. With all of the grandparents present, we revealed her name to everyone. Isla Florence. She was officially no longer "the baby," "they," or even "it." She was a whole person who we all loved immensely. By 8:00 a.m., we were ready to head home from the hospital. Everyone was incredibly happy and in good health, and the three of us were ready to begin life as a new little family.

Overall, my labour was an unexpected and wild experience but for all of the drama it provided, the end result was the birth of our beautiful baby girl, and I wouldn't have it any other way.

About Sara

Sara and her husband Paul are originally from the Hamilton area. She is an elementary school teacher while he is a member of the Canadian Armed Forces. Due to his military career, they currently reside in Petawawa, ON with their daughter and two dogs. Prior to this recent move, they spent two years in Brantford, ON, where their daughter, Isla, was born. They are indebted to the Community Midwives of Brantford for their fabulous care during her birth.

Surprise!

by Sheena McDonald
Toronto, Ontario

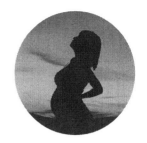

As I sit on my toilet, dazed and confused at the fact that I've just delivered a baby in my apartment, my midwife gently wipes my face. "Is it blood?" I croak.

"No," she replies with a sympathetic smile. "Just some poop."

Let's rewind.

It is eight hours earlier and I bolt upright in bed. Ow. Even though I'm pregnant with my first child, I somehow know in every fibre of my being that it's time.

I shake my partner awake and tell him firmly, "This is it."

"Oh yeah? Okay," he mumbles groggily back. He thinks I mean that this is the very beginning of labour, the minor contractions that will slowly build over many hours. At 40 weeks pregnant, I've had plenty of time to watch countless birth videos on YouTube that show this gradual progression, often transpiring over multiple days.

But that's not what I mean. I'm telling him that *this is happening now*.

It's time to call my midwife and hastily make our way to the birth centre, where I'll ease into an enormous birthing tub and find solace in a quick supply of nitrous oxide.

My midwife arrives about an hour later and performs a quick check to confirm that this is, in fact, happening right now. Her head jerks up in surprise. "You're 10 cm dilated," she exclaims. It takes me a moment to realize that this means I'm fully dilated.

"Listen, it's entirely your call. But how would you feel about doing this here?"

I laugh nervously and glaze around my surroundings – to the dust bunnies, pile of dirty laundry, and general clutter around me.

Then, I imagine delivering my baby in a Honda Fit on the way to the birth centre. "Um, yeah, let's do this," I say.

A flurry of activity follows – the nightstand is cleared to make room for equipment, a plastic covering is draped on the bed, and our two cats are shooed from the bedroom. There's nothing quite like being in the throes of active labour while a cat sniffs your face, I discover.

I soon learn that lying flat on my back in bed makes no sense to my body. No, I need gravity and something to push violently against as the contractions ramp up.

I find myself on my knees and gripping my headboard, screaming through the pain. When I release my death grip, I notice the thick layer of dust that coats the surface, now partially coating my sweaty palms. Mental note: Don't forget to dust the headboard.

There comes a point, as the sun begins to rise, when the pain is so horrific and constant that I don't think I can make it. Does this happen to everyone? A rising panic that you'll die, that your baby will die? That this is it?

"I can't do it!" I scream.

Calmly and confidently, my midwife replies, "But you are. You are doing it."

Thankfully, I'm not doing it alone.

My partner, the one who, just a couple of hours earlier, could barely time a contraction, is now a doula.

He is there, by my side, through it all – feeding me frozen grapes, gripping my lower back during every contraction to help widen my pelvis, and a host of other things I'm unaware of as I travel deeper within myself.

It's time to push and I am now fully in my head, focused on the excruciating task at hand.

I find myself gripping onto the side of my bed while standing in a sort of squat, my legs trembling with the effort of each push. I'm now fully naked and bathed in sweat.

My partner opens the window in the room to let in the fresh spring air and it occurs to me that my neighbours must be waking up to my animalistic howls. I dimly wonder if they'll call the police.

In the end, no one does but I wonder, to this day, if this is something I should be grateful for or concerned about.

My partner is now on the floor below me, prepared to catch the baby. This is it.

An extended scream escapes me, and I feel my baby fully emerge into the hands waiting below.

"Oh my god," my midwife exclaims in amazement. "She's so *big*."

I reach down between my legs and pull up my nine-and-a-half-pound baby girl, a surprise considering that both my partner and I are relatively small people. I weighed a measly five pounds at birth.

I climb gingerly onto the bed and lie down, clutching my giant, slippery, beautiful baby to my chest.

This is only the fourth baby I've ever held in my life.

I don't have a lot of experience with kids. No big extended family with lots of little ones running around, limited babysitting experience, and only a handful of my friends have children so far.

I've never changed a diaper. I don't know what I'm doing.

Yet, I've just climbed Mount Everest and run a marathon. For a moment, I am filled with the knowledge that I am capable of anything. All along, I had a profound inner strength, just waiting to be tapped into.

But I certainly had help.

As my midwife calmly wipes the poop off of my face a short while later (is this poop from the baby? I will never be sure), I am in awe of the physical and emotional support she has just given me. I don't know what to say, how to fully express my gratitude.

Soon, she cheerfully packs her bags and heads off to attend another birth, just another day on the job.

Another mundane miracle awaits.

I tried to articulate my overwhelming feelings over the phone the next day but did not find the words to truly do it justice.

About Sheena

Sheena lives in Toronto with her husband, 2-year-old daughter, and two cats, who get a shout-out in her story. Although she is able to fulfill her love of writing on a daily basis as a communications professional in the non-profit sector, she will seize any opportunity to write creatively.

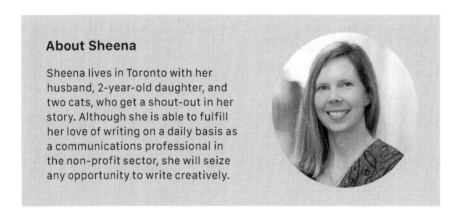

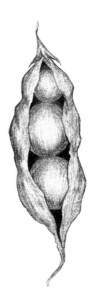

The distinction between pain and suffering is crucial to our understanding of women's emotional wellbeing in labor. ... We postulate that it is not pain, but an inability to cope with pain that is at the root of the concern.

—Penny Simkin, Lisa Hanson, and Ruth Ancheta,
The Labor Progress Handbook, Early Interventions to Prevent and Treat Dystocia

Wednesday's Child

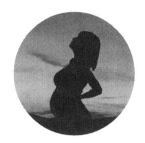

by Sara Wood-Gates
Burlington, Ontario

My water broke at 11 a.m. on a Wednesday. I was on the toilet when I felt the pop and then the whoosh.

Steve and I had been waiting anxiously for something to happen for the last week and a half. He was shipping out to Afghanistan in the next two weeks, no hard date for that either, and we were both hoping for as many days as possible for him to bond with an actual baby rather than a big tummy.

Despite all that waiting, my water breaking was anticlimactic, as I wasn't yet in labour. Not even a twinge. We settled down to lunch after calling the midwives, letting them know what had happened, and hearing that they had finally gotten hospital privileges the day before.

It wasn't until I was in the shower about an hour later that the contractions started. Initially, Steve was timing them for me but as they approached every six minutes within 20 minutes or so, he decided he better have a shower as well if he was going to get one.

Things were progressing quickly.

Our last birthing class, six weeks beforehand, had been an eye-opener for both of us. The teacher had pulled out her trusty 10-centimetre diameter plumbing pipe to show us the size my cervix had to reach to allow the baby to be expelled. I can still feel my jaw dropping, blood draining from my face, as I looked at it. It seemed impossible that a part of my body that had previously held a slim tampon in place, given pleasure to a normal male penis during the creation of the child, could ever accommodate a newborn baby. But I had to put that out of my mind because I had decided on natural childbirth.

That had gone over like a lead balloon with Steve. I believe his exact words were, "I'm a dude and I couldn't even do that." Well, if anything was going to confirm my resolution, those were the words to do it. Hearing his lack of confidence galvanized my resolve. I was going to have a natural childbirth.

By 1 p.m. we were in the car, heading to the hospital. I was in active labour by that time. I wanted to jump out of the car and walk to the hospital rather than suffer the tourniquet that was the seatbelt. As a contraction came on, I twisted to the side, leaning my weight on my hip, rather than take the force of it in a sitting position.

The hospital was only seven minutes away. I thought I would only need to suffer through one contraction before we arrived, but the parking lot was busy that day. As Steve circled the parking lot looking for a good spot, I couldn't stand it in any longer.

"Just find a spot! I don't care where you park!"

Steve checked me into the hospital and then went to move the car from the hash marks he had ended up parking on while I walked to the birthing suite. They tried to get me into a wheelchair, but I was done with sitting. At least with walking, there was a slight distraction from the deep aching that accompanied the contractions. At the time, I wouldn't have described it as pain because it was deeper than that. It was as if I could feel my body physically changing internally with each contraction. It was deeply uncomfortable. However, it had nothing to do with the pain you feel when you cut yourself or sprain an ankle.

Because the midwives had so recently been granted their hospital privileges, I was treated by both them and my doctor. The midwives were an invaluable source of support. They were aware of my desire to proceed naturally, without pain medication of any kind. They ran point for me when I declined medication but was asked repeatedly if I was sure. They got me set up in the room, kept Steve busy, and made me move so my labour would progress.

After arriving and changing into the hospital gown, being checked out internally, and the baby's vitals assessed, the midwives got me back up and walking the halls. Honestly, if I had been left in a room where I was strapped to machines and couldn't do anything but lie there, I likely would have ended up needing some kind of analgesic intervention. Being able to move around was my saving grace.

After being checked again, I was transitioned to the yoga ball. I was sitting on it, leaning on Steve, as wave after wave of contractions crashed over me. At one point, he reached over and rubbed my earlobe as comfort. It felt so loving and reassuring that I tilted my head to the side, capturing his hand between my ear and my shoulder. I was craving more and more comfort. Steve misunderstood and took his hand away. It felt like a warm blanket was being removed, but I was so wrapped up in the intensity of the moment that I couldn't voice my need. There was no space for words.

As things progressed, around 8 cm dilated, they brought me to the tub in the suite. The midwives helped me lower my ungainly body into the water. It was like heaven. As soon as I was immersed, everything became lighter. The water softened the aching, the intensity, and the weight of my body. The relief was instantaneous. I would have stayed in there the entire time, but that hospital didn't allow water births.

Back in the bed, another internal check and I was close to 10 cm. There happened to be a class of paramedics doing their practicum in the hospital and the instructor asked if they could stay for the birth. At that point, I wouldn't have cared if they toured all of Pembroke through the hospital. They phrased it as "showing the paramedics a normal, natural birth." I remember my response was, "There's nothing normal or natural about this!" I think they stayed.

When it came time to push, the feeling that came over me with that contraction was so powerful, so instinctual, so necessary, that I couldn't do anything but push. It was like a wave that would build inside me. Almost the opposite of throwing up. You can't stop yourself from throwing up, no matter how hard you try. This was exactly the same, except the pressure wasn't to push something out of my mouth but to bear down and push into my own body. I had no control over whether I was going to push or not. My body was pushing because it was time.

Steve says he almost missed the birth because he was outside smoking. He's exaggerating. She didn't come out in one or two pushes. It felt endless and as if time stood still, both incredibly quick and infinitely long. He was shocked when he came back in, and I was pushing. While it was happening, I had no idea who was in the room and who wasn't. Someone was always holding my hand and that was all that mattered.

Toward the end, when my daughter was crowning, the doctor was there, as well as the midwives. He offered to do an episiotomy, as he was worried I was going to tear badly without one. I was happy to agree, and Adrianna was born within two pushes. A quick, final explosion. I have since learned that episiotomies were frowned upon. I was disappointed when they wouldn't give me one when my son was born two years later. I wonder what the midwives thought about it at the time. I was happy as I healed up within the week.

Steve had said there was no way he was going to cut the cord when the baby was born. It was gross and disgusting and why would anyone want to do that? But he was right in there, cutting away when they offered. I had read all about how it was most beneficial to wait until the cord finished pulsating to cut it, even if it took a while, but in all the excitement, I didn't even think about it. I also forgot all about my desire to save the cord blood.

Delivering the placenta happened without my noticing. By that time, I was doing skin-to-skin with the tiny live creature that had just sprung forth from my body. I was in utter disbelief. I was in love. Even as my body shed the built-up adrenaline, as I shook and vibrated in my bed, I didn't pay too much attention. At 4:04 p.m., I had become a mother.

What did get my attention was when the doctor started to sew up the episiotomy. I did not know until then that it wasn't possible to freeze the skin. It was almost more painful than the birth itself. I certainly complained more while he was sewing than I did when I was pushing.

That experience was a turning point in my self-esteem. Being able to manage natural childbirth, while everyone around me doubted that I could do it, changed something. That, combined with having a new person that I was responsible for, put me on a new path. A path that made me realize that I could accomplish things that were hard, that seemed impossible, and that others doubted I could.

I'll never forget those first moments of looking into Adrianna's eyes, the knowledge of galaxies shining back at me. All I could think in those moments was, "Oh, of course. It's you." Because in that moment, it felt like I had known her all my life and had been waiting for her forever.

About Sara

Sara Wood-Gates is a single mother of two children living in Burlington Ontario. She has spent most of her career in various customer service roles from serving in restaurants to planning events to counselling job seekers on their careers. Currently, Sara works as a Pre-Sales Solution Architect for an American company, which has allowed her to work from home since 2013. Sara is excited to draw from her wealth of personal stories as she dabbles in writing.

Labour, Delivery, and a Grateful Grandmother

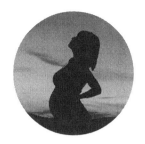

by Sharon Chisvin
Winnipeg, Manitoba

While I knew that I was going to love and adore my grandson from the moment he was born, I never expected that I would have the great privilege of witnessing his birth. But, in response to my daughter and son-in-law's repeated insistence that they wanted me with them during labour and delivery, I made the trip from Winnipeg to Toronto last winter to accompany them to the hospital for a scheduled induction for what an ultrasound had indicated was "a very big baby." My daughter's pregnancy had been easy, but it had followed two miscarriages, and so none of us were taking anything for granted.

Some of the finer details of that day are fuzzy, partly because so much has happened since then (it's been an eventful year for our family and for the world), but this is what I remember.

My daughter had been instructed to be at the renowned downtown hospital at 3 p.m. Thursday, February 14th, but our Uber driver took a surprisingly long time to arrive, was unsure of the best route to the hospital, and seemed stymied by the falling snow and sleet-filled streets. In the end, we arrived at the hospital about 20 minutes late, feeling badly that we may have kept hospital staff waiting.

We need not have worried!

After riding the elevator up the 15th floor, my daughter checked in, completed some paperwork, and was kindly told to wait in the lounge area until a room became available. So, we waited, the three of us excited but calm, and my daughter comfortable and at ease as she watched, with her usual intense interest in people, a parade of expectant women and their partners pace up and down the hallways.

Three hours later, we were escorted to a labour and delivery room, where a nurse told my daughter that the doctor on call, not her regular obstetrician, would be in shortly to begin the induction process. So, we waited, the three of us still excited but calm, although, admittedly, we quickly turned our attention to the door every time we heard footsteps approaching down the hall. Those footsteps did sometimes enter our room, but each time, it was a different nurse, always caring and always friendly, but only there to do a quick check-in and to tell us again that the induction would start soon.

So, we waited, half-heartedly watching videos on my son-in-law's laptop, chatting, reading, snacking, napping, and making a couple phone calls to let family and friends know we were still waiting. Finally, at one in the morning, almost 10 hours after we arrived at the hospital and seven hours after being escorted to the labour and delivery room, the nurses and doctor arrived to begin the induction.

We were all still excited but calm.

As expected, my daughter's contractions came on quickly once her water was broken, and she met their arrival with equal measures of eagerness, fortitude, and fearlessness. Her husband stood by her side, holding one hand, while I stood on the other side, holding the other, and together, we stumbled along, offering her sips of water, encouraging her, praising her, and reminding her to inhale and exhale through the pain. Our efforts were well-intentioned, but they were also unsynchronized, amateurish, and inadequate, and it quickly became apparent to all three of us that we had not prepared for labour as well as we could have. I had clearly relied too much on faded memories of my own labours, some 30 years before, while my daughter and son-in-law, always busy and pulled in many different directions, seemed not to have practised often enough what they had learned in a weekend prenatal class. In the heat of the moment, we also all completely forgot that there was a print-out of helpful breathing exercises tucked into my son-in-law's jeans' pocket.

Three hours after the contractions began, my daughter's resolve and energy were beginning to wane. She requested an epidural, less so because she couldn't manage the pain, but more so because she suddenly began to worry that if the contractions lasted for hours, she would be too exhausted to push when the time came.

I was ushered out of the room when the anesthetist arrived to administer the epidural but invited back in as soon as he left. The three of us slept fitfully then for a couple of hours, waking in the early morning to the news that dilation had barely progressed, and a C-section might be in order. Those words seemed to work a kind of magic, because no sooner were they uttered, then a new check revealed that my daughter was, in fact, fully dilated. It was time to push.

My daughter now laughs when she thinks about what she thought would occur during the pushing phase. A couple strenuous pushes, a few minutes of exertion, and out would come baby! Of course, it wasn't quite like that. There was terrible pain and fatigue. Fleeting flashes of self-doubt. Hand-gripping. Leg holding. Brow wiping. Murmured but ineffective words of encouragement from me and her husband. Worry that the baby may have swallowed meconium. A crowd of nurses, medical students, and specialists gathered around. A head that appeared stuck. A head that had to be suctioned out. A torn cervix from the baby's sunny-side-up exit. A lot of blood. A placenta in pieces. At one point, what I feared was an urgent exchange between the doctor and nurses, but to which my daughter and her husband seemed oblivious. In the end, this beautiful baby boy!

To this day, I do not know if that sense of urgency or concern I thought I overheard between the physician and nurses was real or imagined, but I do know that I held my breath and clutched my daughter's hand—my baby's hand—until I saw the doctor lean away from her, sigh, and say that all was well. By then, the baby—her baby—had been weighed and swaddled (he wasn't "very big" after all), posed for his first photo, and been cuddled by his star-struck father. Perhaps it was then, as the baby was gently placed back into his mother's trembling arms, that my daughter, grateful, enraptured, and in love, began to think that, maybe next time, she, like so many women she knew, would engage the services of a doula.

The next time has come sooner than planned. Just as the playful, curious, and wondrous toddler who has filled my daughter and son-in-law's lives and the life of our entire family with unbounded joy and love, turns 18 months, his baby brother is set to make his entrance. Any day now, in fact.

Despite my daughter's best intentions, there will be no doula at the birth. For just as she was making arrangements for an initial consultation with one in Toronto, COVID-19 came to Canada, and my daughter, son-in law, and grandson hastily packed up and came to Winnipeg to wait out the pandemic. The hoped-for regular face-to-face sessions with a Toronto doula, as a result, never happened, and with all the upheaval and uncertainties that defined the last few months, including new restrictions on how many people could accompany labouring mothers in hospital, my daughter seemed to give up on the doula idea. That is, until someone recently suggested to her that she could engage a doula to do a virtual session.

We just did that online session last week, and though, of course, we know that a single two-hour session cannot replace months of regular face-to-face visits, we feel reasonably confident that we are better prepared for my daughter's second labour and delivery than we were for the first. We certainly know more this time about the various stages of labour, breathing options, massage techniques, and birthing positions, and if we forget what we learned in the excitement of the moment, we will at least remember that we have all this information clearly printed out on handy recipe cards and tucked into my son-in-law's pants' pockets.

I say "we," because at the moment, with COVID-19 in Manitoba reasonably under control, local hospitals are now permitting labouring mothers to be accompanied by two support people, and I am both delighted and honoured to have been invited again to be one of those support people and be present at my daughter's second labour of love.

About Sharon

Sharon Chisvin is a Winnipeg mother of three adult children, and a grateful grandmother who had the privilege of attending the births of all three of her grandsons—in 2019, 2020, and 2021. She works as a journalist, editor, and oral historian, and is the author of the children's picture book, *The Girl Who Cannot Eat Peanut Butter*, and the editor of the *Write to Move* anthology.

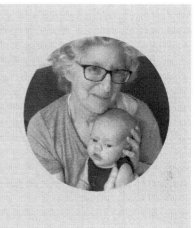

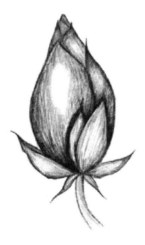

I went into birth uncertain but unafraid. I didn't know what would happen, but I felt prepared, confident that I could birth my child how I wanted. I discovered my body and my daughter had other plans, ones that took me to a dark place where fear and danger took on another dimension. I ended up grateful for the interventions I had not wanted. I didn't necessarily want to learn all of this, but I didn't have a choice.

—**Angela Garbes,** *Like a Mother*

The Dark Road to Life

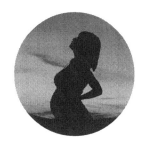

by Mica Pants
South Frontenac, Ontario

I never really thought of myself having kids. I wasn't sure I even liked kids. As far back as I can remember, I have never even held a baby, especially not a wrinkly, translucent, delicate newborn. I did not think they were cute. Moreso, I thought of them as weird looking, with erratic movements. I grew up in big cities, where even at 30, no one I knew had children. No one could afford it. It was like being in your early twenties forever, scrambling to pay rent and living with five other people. My feelings about children and babies never changed, even as my partner of five years started to yearn for a baby. I love Emily. I love Emily and I wanted her to have her dreams. I was indifferent, not opposed. Intuitively, I knew that the challenges I would face as a parent would help my spiritual growth.

When we finally decided to start trying, we had moved from Toronto and had bought a house north of Kingston. We had gotten good stable jobs and our life seemed in order. We were ready. We chose an anonymous donor and went through the Clinical Investigations Unit (thank goodness they changed that name) at Kingston General Hospital. Emily got pregnant on our first try. We felt lucky, golden even.

Emily's pregnancy was typical until the end, but I'll get there. What I want to talk about first is bonding. Not being the gestational parent, the baby and I would not be biologically related, and I was worried about forming a bond and feared that it would feel like Emily's baby and not mine. My sister, during her pregnancy, told me she had heard about a lesbian couple who could share the breastfeeding role by inducing lactation in the non-gestational mother. It sounded so cool. I really wanted to do it and I did. I have to be honest; it was a *lot* of work.

I won't get into details of the process of inducing lactation because that's a long story, but I will mention some challenges that I faced that, maybe, could help medical professionals who might have patients looking to induce in the future. My family doctor had no idea of the process but was happy to prescribe me the necessary medication. I saw a lactation consultant who had no idea of the process but was happy to explain to me the ins and outs of breastfeeding. Our midwives directed me to a protocol online of how to induce lactation but couldn't help me beyond that, as their patient was Emily and the baby, not me.

I was on my own and I did it on my own. It required that I start pumping milk a few months before the due date, every four hours every day. This made for awkwardness at work, for sure, but I was unapologetic about it, and nobody gave me any negative feedback. Most people thought it was cool. I remember feeling so tired because I had to get up in the night to pump. I look back at that time with humour, as I had not yet known how little sleep my future would entail.

As I said before, Emily's pregnancy was typical, until near the end. She started to have low platelet levels and we were worried about having to transfer to the high-risk pregnancy unit from our midwives, as well as some of the complications that could occur, such as pre-eclampsia. We were told that if Emily didn't give birth within a week, she should be induced. We took our midwife on the offer to do a cervical sweep and hoped that she would go into labour soon. Lucky for us, it worked, and in the middle of that night, Em started to have contractions and thought her water broke.

The next day was a blur. I know that we stayed at home most of the time Em was in labour, but beyond that, I can't recall anything until we started having visitors in the evening. Emily's mom, sister, and dad were present. Our midwife showed up and advised Emily to walk to get the labour going. The main floor of our house is connected in a complete circle, almost. Our living room goes into our dining room, then into our kitchen, then into a second living room, and then the circle starts again. Round and round she went, and I followed, and our husky, Chili, followed me. Every few minutes, Em would have a contraction and lean against something. My job was to put pressure on her back at those moments. This was fun and felt magical. The CBC Radio program, "The Signal," was playing. I loved it and would listen to it at work when I used to work overnights. It is now off the air. The labour was probably the last time I heard it. I was excited and loved being at our house during that time. It was comforting.

Our midwife couldn't get reception on her cell since we live in a forested ravine. She had to drive up to the road to make a call, which was kind of funny. However, that was the defining moment that compelled us to get a landline.

It was probably around 11 p.m. when our midwife said we were ready to transfer over to the hospital. Driving was weird and Emily found it hard to have contractions while in the car. It was dark on the country roads with no other cars in sight. The darkness is what I find most unsettling about not being in the city anymore. We coasted through town and parked the car. We made it up to a big room designed for birthing. I set up the birthing playlist we made together, which was mostly meditation music. Em liked this Indigenous flute player R. Carlos Nakai, and a playlist that I found for dog relaxation. We dimmed the lights and continued. Em's sister was the only other person with us. She took a lot of great pictures and was supportive throughout.

I was still pumping every three to four hours, and in retrospect, I realize I was so diligent about it because it was something that I could control. Everything else about having this baby was up to Emily.

Em's pain was getting worse, and she opted to take a hot shower, which she said helped a lot. When she had contractions, she looked like she was in so much pain and her mind was somewhere far away. At this point, she wasn't able to communicate with me that much and I was just trying to guess what she needed. I went in the shower with her for quite a while but decided to leave because I was freezing. This is the one time when I felt I let Emily down. I think she wanted me to stay but was unable to voice it. She came out about 20 minutes later and said she couldn't handle the pain anymore and wanted an epidural.

She said she tried but couldn't do it. I know that she felt guilty for making this decision. We both wanted to have a natural birth. I am positive she felt like she let me down. I think I was supportive in the moment, but it was a sad time because we both thought we had failed the other person. There was an energetic shift at this moment when things went from an idealized birth to something much bleaker.

It felt so long before the anesthesiologist came to do the epidural. It was probably seven or eight in the morning. You could see that the sun had risen through the low windows. She made some quip about "how nice the music was." This aggravated me. It made things seem less magical and more medical. After the epidural, Em felt so much better, and we were advised to rest. We slept for a few hours. When we got up again, Em had dilated enough, and it was time to push.

At some point, out of nowhere, our midwife, who's been caring for us for months, told us she had to leave because she had been up more than 24 hours and it wasn't safe for her to be there anymore. This came so out of the blue; it almost felt like a betrayal. I wish she had warned us of this possibility before the birth. I understand the logic but learning about it two seconds before it happened was a shock.

Two other midwives came in to replace her and went through the pushing part of the labour. Em was lying in the bed with her legs spread and pushed as hard as she could for what seemed like 20 or so rounds. Everybody was so encouraging towards her, but you could see that something was off. The midwives looked worried. Our baby's heartbeat was lowering. Supposedly, our baby was right there and just needed to get past the last hurdle and out into our world. The midwives called on some specialists and 10 or so people came in. They just continued praising and encouraging Em. She had no idea that everyone's faces were serious and worried.

She pushed like a champion. Multiple people tried forceps and there was blood everywhere. I was worried, scared, and felt bad for Em.

They took her away from me for an emergency C-section. They gowned me up and had me sit out in the hall for what felt like an eternity on a cold metal stool. Our midwife wasn't recognizable in the sea of blue gowns and face masks, but she took our camera and said she would get some good shots. I started crying and I couldn't stop. I didn't know why, and two years later, I still don't. The other midwife tried to comfort me, but I was not into it. How could they split us up?

When they finally let me in, I rushed in to be with Emily. It felt as though she was strapped to the table. She saw that I was upset and tried to comfort me. I should have been the one comforting her. I, once again, felt like I failed her. Whatever they were doing started to make her whole body convulse and she vomited off to the side. The anesthesiologist caught her vomit and was kind to her. This was horrible to watch, and I was not sure what I was supposed to do.

There was a curtain blocking Em's view beyond her breasts. I found our camera discarded. The replacement midwife was busying around being useful. There were at least 15 blue gowned people running around, doing important things. I took some pictures and was just in time as they raised our baby out of Em's belly. His eyes were wide open, and he looked confused. He did not cry. He was a boy. This also shocked me. I had made myself believe since day one that we were having a girl. My intuition was wrong and that pained me. They did all of their tests as quickly as possible, and the midwife handed him over to me. I was not thrilled. I just wanted to be with Emily. I was the first of us to hold him and the midwife showed me how to get him to latch. This should have been a beautiful moment in the midst of all the chaos. I had worked hard to induce lactation, and we had carefully planned this unique moment when I would breastfeed him for the first time, but I didn't want any of it. I was tired. I was sad. I just wanted to be with Emily.

We shuffled into a recovery room, and I finally got to pass him over to Emily. She looked so proud and happy. It was a relief. It made me feel way better. This was her dream, and I was happy to be part of it. The heavy emotions, drama, and lack of sleep settled, and we switched to our roles of being new moms.

About Mica

Mica Pants (he/him), is a queer trans artist from South Frontenac County, Ontario. He is passionate about art, energy work, and spirituality. He has spent over a decade hustling in the social services and has recently carried and birthed the newest addition to his family. He has not written about it yet.

Follow his @micapantsart or www.micapantsart.com

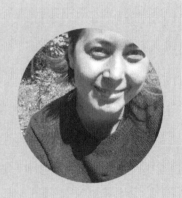

The Middle Child

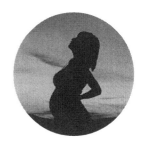

by Gretchen Huntley
Kingston, Ontario

Having child number one was normal as can be
As a matter of fact, so was number three
Now number two was different; let me tell you why
That kid came into the world practically on the fly

It was very early in the morn when I actually awoke
My pains were five minutes apart; that was not a joke
Now I should have thought about it as it was number two
But for some strange reason I wasn't sure what to do

You see my first was slow and steady,
There was lots of time to get ready
There was no whirlwind or frantic flurry
Number one was in no hurry
But apparently number two didn't think the same
And hurry up, don't waste time, seemed to be her game
So when I woke at 8 a.m., it took me by surprise
Could this kid be on the way as I'd barely opened my eyes?

So, I called my friend who was a nurse
Not sure if that helped or made it worse
She acted like I had no brain
I had called her so I shouldn't complain

"Get to the hospital," she said, "right now!"
Boy, she was snippy, I thought, holy cow

So off we went to the KGH
but had to make one stop
It slowed us down a little bit;
I thought my belly would pop
Now the pains, they just kept a-coming
Coming really fast
I wondered if we'd get there in time,
I was sure I wouldn't last
We pulled into the hospital as the clock struck 10 a.m.
I sighed with great relief and then I said, "Amen"

Now the nurse acted like
I was being a whiny little shrew
Until she peered between my legs
And there was you-know-who
The nurse took another look
As I tried hard to be brave
She rolled her eyes and said I guess
We'll have to forego the shave
And that was when it happened
I gave the nurse a bath
Water gushed everywhere
For a moment, I thought I might laugh

She left that room like a bat out of hell
And returned with a doctor who seemed kind of swell
He was good looking, but I didn't care
As long as he concentrated on that baby down there

He delivered my little girl quicker than a wink
The time was ten after ten,

THE MIDDLE CHILD

Well, that is what I think
He stitched me up
And leaned on my knees
Said, "Well, that job is done"
And he really looked pleased

He gave me a smile and walked out the door
Leaving me with a butt that was really sore
And a sweet little girl I named Tina Louise
A beautiful baby to kiss and to squeeze

My baby arrived on a very special date
Some would say that it was fate
I lost my daddy many years ago
On the very same month and day
And now because of my little girl
That sadness has melted away

About Gretchen

Gretchen Huntley is an author from Kingston. She wrote three children's books, as well as a book on her son's journey with cancer. She is the founder of The Get-Well Gang, a group of crafters who make and donate 100% cotton caps to cancer patients.

During the beginning of COVID-19, she turned to poetry to help her through the dark times. The outcome was a small poetry book called *Reality and Me*.

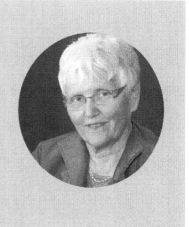

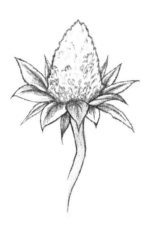

The most common way people give up their power is by thinking they don't have any.

—Alice Walker

Oliver's Birth

by Anne-Marie Laplante
Kingston, Ontario
Vancouver, British Columbia

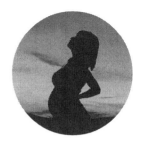

Oliver's Birth on April 21st, 2008, I was blessed with a lovely home VBAC (vaginal birth after cesarean) of my baby boy, Oliver. This is our story.

Oli's 4-year-old brother Sam was born in May 2005 at St. Paul's Hospital in Vancouver B.C., after an uneventful pregnancy. However, it was a complicated, stressful, and long labour, ending in a cesarean following failed forceps. I often joke (somewhat) that I had experienced almost every complication during his birth. A classic cascade of interventions, including induction at 42+2 days past due, epidural, oxytocin, maternal fever, heart rate decelerations, exhaustion, and a baby boy who was born angry at the world, having endured such a stressful welcome. While I recovered from surgery, Sam spent a few hours in the NICU after being resuscitated. It was hours before I saw him, and I'd always felt cheated at not having been there to hold him during his first hours.

In a weird and fateful twist of events during my year of maternity leave, I was offered a position as the office manager at Pomegranate Community Midwives, and soon learned that such birth experiences—while certainly not all negative—are, unfortunately, more common than I had thought in hospital settings.

When I became pregnant with Oli, I hoped this experience would be different. Better. Luckily for us, our midwives were also our friends, so it was easy to convince my husband, Neil, that it would be best for us to birth at home. I spent the next few months telling everyone that we were hoping for a home birth, but I knew full well that, sometimes, things are beyond our control; mamas get tired, labour takes too long, babies just don't want to be born at home, and you might have to make the difficult decision to transfer to the hospital to birth your baby. Since I also had the risks of a VBAC to consider, I knew that the stars needed to align for Oli's birth to go according to our plan. I knew the risks and the rewards of both birth locations, yet deep down, I so very much wanted this baby to be born at home.

Starting at 37 weeks, I did a lot of labour prep in hopes of not going late again. I began weekly, then twice weekly acupuncture sessions, drank a lot of birthing tea, took evening primrose oil caplets, and did everything else my midwives and doula suggested.

At approximately 39 weeks, I started experiencing mild contractions on and off for the weekend. I continued with my days spending my time shopping, going out for lunch, and resting with friends and family. The contractions were coming every 20 minutes or so. I was able to walk through them, breathing and distracting myself. On Friday and Saturday night, at the suggestion of my midwives, I took a warm bath, some Tylenol and Gravol, and had a good night's sleep. However, by Sunday morning, I was tired of niggling and wanted to get things going. I went to an acupuncture session I had previously booked and hoped I would meet my baby soon.

That night, while my husband was getting Sam ready for bed, my contractions suddenly picked up in strength and intensity. My husband came down to the living room at 8:30 p.m. and found me in tears on my hands and knees. Initially, I was scared. I had been dealing so well all weekend, and though I had wanted this so badly, I was afraid of the sudden intensity of the pain. Could I really do this? Neil ran a warm bath for me, and the water felt wonderful, but the contractions continued. Every time a contraction began, I would curl over on my side, close my eyes, and moan. Neil grew nervous, asking if I needed our doula Aleksandra to come, and if we needed to page the midwives.

It's interesting to me that, even in the midst of labour, I worried about what I was supposed to sound like – what were those guttural sounds I was supposed to be doing? Was I breathing right? Was I labouring correctly? At 9 p.m., the intensity increased enough that my husband called Aleksandra, who arrived shortly after. Contractions were coming every two to three minutes, lasting 60 seconds. The three of us laboured together for about two hours in the bath, then walking around our house while Aleksandra offered encouragement and sips of water, and Neil held my hand through contractions.

I once read in a blog that, during labour, I can expect to "grunt and sweat and pant and push and poop and moan and rock, and I will probably even barf. This is what it will take to get my baby out, and this is okay. I don't have to like it. I just have to do it." This particular passage resonated with me, and it mirrors how I saw my experience. I vocalized a lot during labour: yelled, moaned, cried, and just let myself be in the moment. Let myself be scared yet strong in the comfort of my home, surrounded by people who loved me.

Sensing that labour was coming along quickly, Aleksandra paged our midwife at 11 p.m. and she arrived a few minutes later. By this time, I was walking around our house, working to get Oli in the best position possible by doing lunges, squats, and leaning into Neil whenever a contraction would hit. Immediately upon arriving, Janice listened to Oli's heartbeat, and everything sounded great! At 11:50 p.m., while sitting on the toilet, labouring, my water broke with a pop and a gush. This is one of my most vivid moments in my labour and it coincides with when I hit transition. I remember losing control and looking into the toilet to see if the fluid was meconium-stained (which might have necessitated a transfer to the hospital). I also remember Janice saying to me, "You're in transition!" and I thought, of course, I am! This makes much more sense and totally explains why I'm having a hard time coping.

At this time, there was a bit of flurry to get me to the couch, since Janice hadn't even had a chance to check me to see how dilated I was – 9.5 cm! I was in shock, and I remember laughing when she told me that. I knew then that I could do this.

While I continued to labour with Neil at my side, Aleksandra filled the birth pool, and Janice called for backup. Once my urges to push got stronger, I started pushing in the pool, alternating between floating on my back and squatting, holding on to Neil for support. I pushed like this for an hour but couldn't quite get enough of a grip for the pushes to be effective enough. At 1:40 a.m., I got out of the tub and sat on the birthing stool, and that's where I really felt myself pushing. Pushing was, by far, the strangest and most powerful sensation of my entire labour. It felt out of control – my whole body pushing, every fibre, every muscle working to get this baby out.

Not long after I sat on the birthing stool, our "little" 9-pound Oli was born and was immediately placed in my arms, wailing his lungs out. I had done it! Drug-free, complication-free, the way that I had imagined it could be, and the way I had dreamt it would be. We cuddled and bonded, nursed and snacked, while admiring our new baby boy in the quiet and comfort of our living room.

Shortly after, Janice helped me shower, dress, and then she tucked us into bed. I was suddenly exhausted. Oli met his big brother Sam (who had slept through the entire thing) that morning and life continued on as it should. In the end, Oli's birth was a lot easier than I had anticipated, yet much more intense than anything I'd ever experienced, and I will be forever grateful.

"There is a secret in our culture, and it's not that birth is painful. It's that women are strong." - Laura Stavoe Harm

About Anne-Marie

After leaving Ontario at the end of high school for adventures in Montreal, Lake Louise, and Vancouver, Anne-Marie and her husband moved back to Kingston in 2010. While living in Vancouver, she was immensely lucky to have been the office manager at Pomegranate Community Midwives from 2006 to 2010. She remains eternally grateful for everything the community taught her about the strength of women and the power of birth. Her boys are now 11 and 14 years old, and they live in the Skeleton Park neighbourhood.

In Gratitude

by Scarlete Flores-Singh
Kingston, Ontario

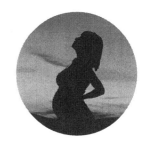

At midnight, our doula, Rachel, rushed to the bath, where I lay helpless. Immediately, she held my hand, and her energy enveloped me in an instant. There was calm as she told me, "It's alright. I'm right here." She squeezed my hand; I squeezed hers back.

My husband, who has been an amazing partner throughout, was on the phone, trying to get a hold of our midwife. I could sense his pulse and his breath quickening as he tried to stay calm. He was pacing to and fro, speaking in a whisper.

I felt the need to scream. The walls around me were too thin; they wouldn't have contained it. My contractions were so strong, it felt like my entire body might explode. Closing my eyes only brought the pain into focus.

Then, I felt my doula's gentle touch.

I looked at her. I stared deeply into her eyes and squeezed her fingers with the strength of a lion. She took it in. My pain travelled from my bump all the way to her hands. She took in so much that she forgot to take off her wedding ring; I nearly crushed it. She took it off.

When our midwife finally arrived, we learned that my daughter was crowning, so we called an ambulance.

Through everything, I wanted to push. I wanted to give birth right there and then. Despite my best efforts to get dressed, my hands kept pulling my pants down.

"I'm doing this here! Now!"

"No, you're not," said my midwife, pulling my pants back up.

I understood. We had planned for a hospital birth for many reasons, including my struggle with mental health. My midwife was right.

My doula, too, was right. She stood by me through it all. Everyone was busy but she focused solely on me. I had her full attention. I think she swallowed all my anxieties, because throughout that night, I felt a sense of calm and peaceful power. All of my fear, all of my insecurity, all of my uncertainty was gone, nowhere to be found.

The ambulance came. I arrived at the hospital with my husband and met her at the doors. We were a good crew. She was on my right side, my husband on my left. Twenty minutes passed and then my daughter, my beautiful angel, arrived at last. She didn't cry for one whole day. She, like me, felt so secure in this world, with these people. My daughter was welcomed by an amazing community and my doula was an integral part of it.

I could never have had such an amazing pregnancy and birth without the help of one of the most empathetic people I know: my doula.

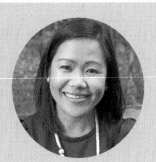

About Scarlete

Scarlete is a mom to an adorable 6-year-old girl. Despite the challenges that came with her pregnancy, recalling her beautiful birth story gives her peace and hope. She wrote this story for her doula, Rachel.

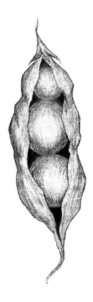

The doula starts out developing a trusting relationship. Soon she becomes a quiet and calming presence. As labor progresses, she moves to a more intense, stronger nurturing role - pacing herself according to the mother's needs and the power of the birth process itself. Her own role with each mother has this developmental aspect and ends with a close tie, for she has shared one of the great moments in a woman's, and a family's life.

- Marshall and Phyllis Klaus, *The Doula Book: How a Trained Labor Companion Can Help You Have a Shorter, Easier and Healthier Birth*

A Doula Letter

by Carrie Allen
for Rebecca Young Family
Canmore, Alberta

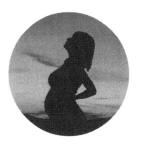

October 15, 2008

Dear Sidney,

The story of your birth is one of great anticipation, intention, love, and joy. Your parents were thrilled about you from the moment they learned of your existence. They took the time during the pregnancy to learn about and plan for your entry into this world, choosing the location and their support team. They wanted to create a naturally beautiful and memorable birth experience. They knew that this day had the potential to be great and powerful, and for them, this meant without question, a birth in the comfort of their own home with the support of a midwife and a doula.

Your due date was October 7th, but your parents were expecting you to arrive later. On Tuesday, October 14th, your mom started feeling mild contractions at around 7 p.m. She had been experiencing Braxton Hicks contractions for several weeks during the night, but something about these contractions on this particular day felt different. At 2:30 a.m. on October 15th, your dad called me to say that your mom was experiencing regular contractions that were about 10 minutes apart and lasting about 20 seconds. Your mom was managing well by breathing through the contractions and rested between them.

By 5 a.m., the intensity had picked up and they were ready for me to come over. Your mom was still managing the contractions while lying on her side on the bed and breathing deeply. She thought it would be best to continue in this position because she was comfortable there and could get some rest.

She feared that she might run out of energy later, but I reassured her that labouring women seem to have an endless supply of energy.

We decided it would be good to try to rest for now but that soon, she would likely need to get up and move around. The contractions were three to five minutes apart, lasting 30-60 seconds. I massaged your mom's hips and reassured her that she was doing well. Your dad lay by her side, his head touching hers while he massaged her arms and whispered gentle words of encouragement. Your dad was becoming excited at the thought of meeting you; he could barely contain his emotion. He would say things like, "We're going to be parents," and "It's really happening." He contacted some friends and family to let them know that your mom was in labour. When I first arrived, your mom showed lots of excitement too, and talked and joked between contractions, but with every progressing contraction, she became more inwardly focused.

At 6:45 a.m. your mom decided to try a different position, so we went downstairs, and she sat on the ball and ate a few spoonfuls of cereal. She found the ball uncomfortable, and after about a half hour, decided to go back on her side on the bed. At 8:15 a.m., the contractions were getting noticeably stronger. I encouraged your mom to make deeper sounds, more like groaning or humming. At 8:45 a.m., your mom said she felt a pop inside and thought her water broke. She decided to get up, and sure enough, it had ruptured. Mireille, your midwife, arrived just seconds later. She checked your mom and found that she was 4-5 cm dilated, but you were still high up. She suggested getting up and letting gravity and movement assist in the progression of labour. Your dad and I helped your mom get dressed and we headed out the door for a walk. The contractions were getting more intense and closer together, so we didn't walk too far; just down the driveway and past a couple of houses. It was a beautiful, sunny morning but cool, and your mom, who had been warm in the house, was now getting chilled. When we went back inside, your mom immediately went on all fours on the bottom of the staircase. She laboured there for several contractions until she started to feel a lot of pressure. We moved to the bathroom, where she laboured on the toilet for several more contractions until the pressure progressed to an urge to push. I thought to myself, *could she really be fully dilated already?* Mireille asked your mom to walk back upstairs to the bed, where she would check to see the progression. Afterwards, she said, "Your baby's right there!" and so, your mom reached down to feel the top of your head. Nurse Deb arrived moments later and became the final addition to your mom's support team.

At 10:30 a.m., your dad got a warm bath ready, and your mom got in. She tried several positions, initially leaning forward on all fours, then lying back, and finally, squatting with your dad supporting her from behind. Your mom expressed frustration at how long the pushing stage was taking. However, things were progressing at a good pace for a first-time labour. At times, your mom questioned whether she could push you out. She needed to know that you were moving down and would eventually be born. Several times, your mom was encouraged to reach down and touch your head so that she could see for herself that you were moving down. Your dad, Mireille, Deb, and I echoed each other's words of encouragement to help your mom remain strong. Once given this reassurance, that we believed she could do it, she regained her confidence and pushed with such concentration, focus, and determination. She would recite phrases like, "I can do this," "I am strong," "Yes," and "Open." Deb read aloud some positive affirmations that your mom had posted on the bathroom mirror.

At 11:15 a.m., your mom started to feel the burning sensation that happens near the end of the pushing stage. We were all getting excited as we started to see the top of your head emerging. Your mom continued pushing with Mireille guiding her to do it slowly. Once again, your mom moved into a semi-reclined position, and at 11:47 a.m. on Wednesday, October 15th, you were born into the warm water. With the assistance of Mireille, your dad caught you, lifted you out of the water, and placed you in your mother's arms. Your parents welcomed you into the world with smiles, tears, and words of love. As they gazed upon you for the first time, they were filled with wonder, amazement, and joy. It was amazing to witness this moment.

This was a day your parents will never forget; a day that started with great anticipation and excitement; a day that required immense emotional and physical strength; a day that was filled with devotion, affection, and continuous support; a day that ultimately filled your parents' hearts with immense love and pure joy. This was the day you were born.

When I reflect upon your birth, the words "trust," "believe," "determination," and "love" come to mind. Your parents chose their support team carefully and placed their trust in us. Everyone present trusted in the birth process and believed in your mom's ability to birth you naturally. Your dad's deep love and admiration for your mom enabled him to be attentive to her physical and emotional needs. He knew what was important to her and remembered her wishes. He continuously reminded her how strong she was and how much he believed in her. He reminded her of the support of her friends and family, the letters they wrote, and the strand of beads they made in her honour. Your dad was continuously present with your mom, breathing and humming along with her. Your mom trusted her body and believed in her inner strength; she knew exactly what to do. All she needed was encouragement to continue doing it. She worked with such strength, focus, and determination to bring you into this world. With the start of each contraction, you could sense that she was working to push negative thoughts away and replace them with positive ones that allowed her to stay strong and focused. She would gain her strength from the four of us who supported her and from deep within herself while she moved through each contraction. It was inspiring to watch. There is no doubt that your mom experienced intense discomfort, but her determination and her love for you allowed her to fulfill her desire to birth you naturally. The moment that you stared into your parents' eyes for the very first time, love enveloped the three of you.

I am so grateful that I was invited to share in the journey of your birth. It was truly a wondrous occasion. May you have love, faith, trust, and determination to guide you throughout your life.

Love your doula,

Carrie Allen

About Carrie

This letter was written by our doula, Carrie Allen, after our daughter's birth in Canmore, Alberta. I have Carrie's permission to include the letter in this book. The letter was part of Carrie's doula package, and we had no idea how special it would be to have such a wonderful gift. It was so special, in fact, that we asked the doulas at our following two births here in Ontario to write letters as well, so now, each one of our kids has one. It's hard to find the words to describe how supported I felt from all of our doulas before, during, and after our births. Here's to all the birthing mommas who have a doula as part of their support team.

My Mom Job Journey

by Bonnie Jean-Louis
Hawkesbury, Ontario

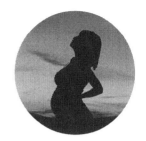

It all started in 1981, when my mother (who had been malnourished and abused as a child) was pregnant with me and confined to a bed for hours, hooked up to an electronic fetal monitor (EFM), and coerced to accept an epidural she never asked for. An episiotomy and forceps were used to deliver me, cone head and all, because they thought my heart decelerated alarmingly while making my way through the birth canal. Little did they know back then, that even though EFM was a great new tool, it was not necessarily accurate. As a big baby, I had to make my way through a passage that was probably stricken with rickets, and constricted by the supine position she was kept in.

Nonetheless, I was born alive, my mom survived, and my family was grateful for the doctor's work, even though it left my mom emotionally and physically scarred for the second time. All the confidence she could ever have gained had been taken away from her. She had a traumatic birth that could be called obstetrical violence today. What would have happened if she would have been given a different birth environment? Probably a wonderful start into motherhood.

My mom got over most of her fear and gave birth to my sister five years later. She took this opportunity to give me the whole shebang of sexual education. My sister was born four days prior to my birthday by C-section because she was breech. My mother always thought her C-section was destiny so that she would not have to go through another bad vaginal birth experience. She was thankful until C-section complications arose. For a few days, they would tell her that the after-pain was normal, even though she knew something was wrong. It took the medical team five days to realize that she had a football-sized hematoma formed in her uterus. She needed another surgery to drain the excess blood. She came out of the hospital three weeks after my sister and was in bedrest for three months. This experience was probably as traumatic as the first one, but only she knows. She is still fearful of doctors today, and who can blame her? Still, she believes they saved her life, and that birth should happen in a hospital.

At 15 years old, I was diagnosed with a severe scoliosis in my lower back and was told I might never be able to bear children. As is often the case with scoliosis, the cause was unknown, but they are sometimes caused by a forceps' extraction at birth.

I was a bit depressed by this state of affairs and was stricken by lower back pains. However, I finished my college education and made a successful career as a photographer and international development worker.

In 2001, I met the traveling photographer-author-midwife Muriel Bonnet del Valle, creator of the book *La naissance, un voyage*. She talked about the different ways of birthing around the world, and the idea that fear is the biggest inhibitor to natural birthing. This idea is emphasized through the work of French physician, Frédérick Leboyer, who advocated for natural births, and the work of French obstetrician, Michel Odent, who favoured water births. I was mesmerized and inspired. I had hoped to carry a child one day, but I also knew that I had a lot of work to do mentally to overcome my own fears about childbirth.

Finally, in 2007, I became pregnant with my son, and I immediately secured a midwife. I decided to have a hospital birth, but because our midwife did not have privileges at the closest hospital to us, we would have to make the drive to Montfort Hospital instead.

When the day finally came, we drove an hour and a half in morning traffic, hoping not to give birth on the side of the road. At the hospital, I laboured in the water, and it worked best to ease my back pain. As soon as my water broke, my midwife emptied the bath. My midwife was amazing, and she advocated for me with the ward doctors because they had thought they should intervene. However, I was firm that as long as my life and my baby's life were safe, I did not want any interventions. After 12 hours of labour, along with an anterior lip of the cervix at 10 cm for a few hours, I gave birth to my 9 lbs, 1 oz son in the squat position. There were lots of tears, but the hard work had finally come to an end. In the end, I discovered that it was the birth I wanted.

All through my pregnancy, I prepared for the birth, but I did not prepare for the fourth trimester. At home with my newborn, breastfeeding was the next challenge. I knew I was going to succeed, but what a hard job it was! It took three weeks of no sleep and pumping around the clock (without ever being able to sit straight, as I had suffered a tear that needed healing). I would fall asleep in the tub while pumping, and my sister or partner would finger feed my son until, finally, he latched on successfully.

Yes! Finally! Unfortunately, the challenges didn't end there.

My son's epiglottis wasn't closed properly, so he threw up a lot at every feeding until he was 8 months old. With this condition, it was hard for me to leave the house, and so, the isolation inevitably led to my depression. I often say it took me close to five years to catch up on the energy lost of those first few years after my firstborn. If anyone had asked me if I wanted another child, there would have been no hesitation; "Hell no!"

Sure enough, in 2016, we were surprised with a second pregnancy. Nine years after my first pregnancy, I had hoped things would have changed. Back then, my midwife had worked hard to gain hospital privileges. However, it was still hard to find a midwife who could attend me all the way in Hawkesbury. I called every midwife clinic and birth centre, asking to be put on waitlists, when, at 32 weeks into my pregnancy, I finally got a call offering me the care I was hoping for.

Once again, I read all the books and opted to have a water birth. My partner prepared well for this experience too. Then, on my partner's birthday, I went into labour. My contractions started at around 6 a.m. At 9:30 a.m., we were having coffee on the front porch with friends who were visiting from

Quebec City. After another hour of irregular contractions that lasted 8 to 15 minutes, they finally settled to two-minute intervals.

I called the on-call midwife, who said that I may have to go to the birth centre. I knew there was no way I was going to make the hour and a half drive there, so the midwife recommended I get into my birthing pool and see if things would calm down or speed up. Once in the tub, I knew there was no way I would ever get out of there. No way was I heading up to Ottawa, even if it meant delivering my baby with the local paramedics instead of a midwife.

Thankfully, an hour later, the midwife arrived from the city. My partner said goodbye to our visiting friends and jumped in the pool with me. When I explained to my midwife that I had a severe scoliosis, she showed my partner how to do hip squeezes. That comfort measure was a savior. I came to understand later that my scoliosis had paralyzed my lower back while I was in labour. Being in the tub made all the difference in the world. I prepared well for my pregnancies, but nothing could have prepared me for this paralyzing sensation.

Instead of hating myself for not being able to move around, or being fearful of what was happening, I embraced the opportunity of floating while my partner and doula would rotate me in the water from time to time. If my partner was busy during a contraction, I would be in agonizing pain but someone else would pitch in, and then I could breathe and relax through my rushes once again.

Three hours later, I felt the urge to push. I wanted to avoid another third-degree tear, so I chose to trust my body and I followed my own rhythm. Suddenly, I felt the ring of fire and I appreciated that my body was telling me how close we were. I embraced the opportunity to feel my daughter's head as it made its way through. After 10 minutes of pushing, I reached down and caught my baby girl.

At 3:37 p.m. (the hour of my own birth) on the 20th of August (my partner's birthday), our 8 lbs, 14 oz daughter was born in the comfort of our own home. Two hours later, I was being fed a nourishing meal, my baby was sleeping, and we were left in our bed to cuddle and bond.

What a difference between my mom's experience of giving birth and my second birth; such a long journey to change fear and powerlessness into confidence and empowerment from one generation to the next.

I now wish that type of transcendence in birth to every birthing person out there, as I've felt, seen, and been proven it can affect so many spheres in life. Every woman, child, family, and community, deserves such a paradigm shift of the modern birth culture.

About Bonnie

Bonnie Jean-Louis is the founder of The Mom Job - Univers Mamans. She is an experienced professional Photographer and Community Health Coordinator and she is also a certified Labour, Birth and Postpartum Doula, Perinatal Educator, PAIL Advocate and Birth Photographer.

Bonnie is passionate about providing adequate evidence-based holistic moral support, the right to choose one's primary care providers and preferred birth place, while rethinking and advocating for The Mom Job.

You can follow her at @universmamans on Instagram or at https://www.facebook.com/universmamans or call 613-494-5007, to access our free phone service to discuss with a doula.

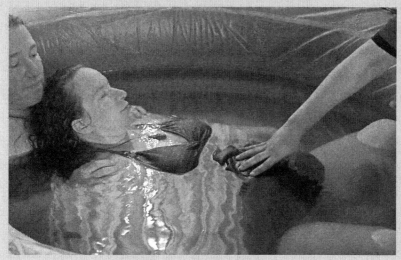

Photography: Stéphane Hunter. Used with permission.

Curbside Delivery

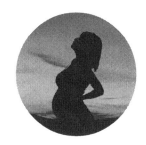

by Sabrina Malach
Toronto, Ontario

On Thursday, May 21st, 2020, there was a spectacular sunrise over Toronto's skyline. I briefly witnessed it from the backseat of the car as we zoomed along Highway 401. I squatted on all fours, trying my best not to birth our child in the back seat of the car. It was 5:45 a.m., and I had spent the last five and half hours labouring at home.

My precipitous labour was unusually quick for a first pregnancy. As we were in the midst of COVID-19, our midwife wasn't able to come into our house, so we weren't clear on how fast things were progressing. When my contractions came on hard and fast, all the plans I made for a long, candlelit, meditative birth with back rubs while sipping bone broth were thrown out the window.

There is a Yiddish proverb that we know well; *Der mentsh trakht un got lakht* (Man plans, and God laughs). I've come to understand the importance of flexibility and change, and to be adaptable in times of crisis. From the beginning, the pandemic demanded that we alter our plans, including going to medical visits without the father, walking into buildings full of masked folks, and not being able to have the midwife in our home during labour and after the birth. All of that was unsettling. Bringing a new life into the world during this pandemic was complicated. I kept thinking to myself, *what kind of future are we walking into? Is it fair to create life on a planet full of viruses, climate catastrophes, corruption, greed, and racism?* The coronavirus seemed to add yet another layer to the laundry list of hardships this and future generations will have to bear.

Just before midnight, I began to feel cramping, and I knew that the journey into early labour had begun. As this was my first pregnancy, we anticipated a long labour, which is the norm for most first-time births. Never one to follow convention, when I felt the overwhelming urge to push only a few hours later, we understood that we were in a unique and urgent situation. By 5:50 a.m., there was no doubt the baby was on her way.

The father and his 19-year-old daughter helped me on what seemed like a marathon trek, as I attempted to walk to the car with what felt like a softball coming out of my vagina. I thought I might be crowning, but hoped I was wrong. I crawled into the back of the car and got on all fours while the daughter's father rubbed my back. Amidst my moans and groans, I screamed, "I'm crowning!" I looked up, noticing the spectacular rays of an early May morning, and I could tell we were moving eastbound. He quickly responded, "Hold on, honey, we are almost there," while hoping that I was misusing the term "crowning" and that our baby wasn't that close to joining us. I didn't think I could hold her in any longer, let alone long enough to arrive at the hospital. When I found the strength to peer up yet again and saw the brilliant sun, I became exceedingly aware of my power and the beauty of life. That awareness calmed me enough to keep the baby inside for a few more minutes.

When we finally arrived at the hospital, the father bolted from the car and scrambled to find the entrance amid the maze of locked doors due to COVID-19. He was screaming, "Help us! We're having a baby!" His daughter helped me crawl out of the car. In a stroke of profound instinct, where all logic, self-consciousness, and insecurity disappeared, I exited the car, stripped off all my clothes, spread my legs, and demanded, "Get behind me and catch the baby." With one swift and powerful push, our beautiful baby girl was born and caught by her older sister in the parking lot of North York General Hospital as the sun rose to welcome her to Earth.

Acting without any prior knowledge, the baby catcher feared that her seconds-old, cone-head, purple, quiet sister was not okay. When the baby finally cried, she instinctively passed her blood-and-poop-covered sibling, who was still attached to the umbilical cord, through my legs, and I blissfully held her on my naked body.

The father, who had left two girls in the car only moments before, returned and saw, to his wonder, the new mom, standing broadly in the open air, naked and full of blood, holding their new baby girl in her arms. The sun's rays shone upon them all.

Only moments later, our calls for help were finally answered. Sixty medical staff flooded to the scene. It was a "Code Pink" with all hands on deck. As they lay me down in my oxytocin-blissed-out-joy, I looked up at all the masked faces and saw the kindness in all of their eyes. I felt safe, supported, and cared for as our baby girl lay on my chest, both of us covered in diverse bodily fluids and membranes, surrounded by a team of loving healthcare workers.

My midwife pushed her way through the masked crowd, and I was surprised I could recognize her behind her mask and scrubs. "Is that you?" I asked. I cried, reassured that she was there, as she cut the cord that had bound me to my girl for the previous nine months. The midwife and the father took my daughter inside to warm her up while I remained on the concrete to ensure I didn't hemorrhage. A few minutes later, we were reunited inside the hospital. New rules had it that Daddy was only allowed to stay with us for three hours, after which he had to leave.

Soon after, I had to take a COVID-19 swab. This experience was almost as painful as the labour itself. It seemed torturous to me, after having such an epic labour, to have a swab stuck so far up my nose, it hit my forehead. Throughout my 24 hours at the hospital, I experienced how the pandemic was impacting the birthing wards. Nurses would check in on us behind Plexiglass shields, and mothers had to spend the first 24 hours alone with their babies without the support or visits of family members. Despite these protocols, the moments were still so precious. Over those 24 hours, I got to intimately bond with my daughter, and I felt deeply cared for by the nurses, even though I couldn't even see their faces.

Despite having a baby in the parking lot during a pandemic, I will never forget the kindness of the hospital staff, my raw and ancient instinct, and the power and beauty of the sunrise on that unforgettable morning.

This morning, I watched the sunrise over Lake Simcoe with our 5-week-old daughter. As our eyes locked, I reminded her that her name, Mira Orli, was inspired in part by that radiant sun. In Hebrew, *Mira* means "the one who shines," and *Orli* means "my light," a living reminder of the beautiful star that gives us all life. It was that light that distracted me long enough so that she would be born under the sunshine in the parking lot of North York General Hospital and gave birth to a whole new meaning to "curbside delivery."

About Sabrina

Sabrina Malach is a lifelong environmental advocate working in urban agriculture and pollinator conservation. She is a beekeeper and an urban farmer, and her sweetest harvest is the birth of her beautiful daughter, Mira Orli. Sabrina lives in Toronto.

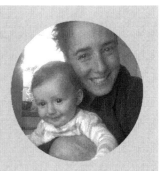

After Hours

by Jennifer Osmond
Clarenville, Newfoundland-Labrador

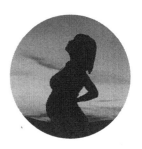

The summer air was cool, the heat from the day drifting away as the moon took over from the sun in the sky. The night was black, the darkness pierced by the headlights of a red 2002 Subaru that hurtled down the highway, breaching the speed limit.

Behind the wheel, white-knuckled, and still half asleep from being awoken from a post-night-shift nap, Andrew drove on. Beside him, Jennifer's rounded belly betrayed the reason for their haste. She was five days past her due date and had just finished putting her nearly 3-year-old daughter to bed a mere hour before – her daughter's last night as an only child. Jennifer realized the significance of that statement in the back of her mind, but it was almost too good to be true that this day was finally here. Another tightening had her squeezing her eyes shut and she practiced the breathing exercises taught to her in the birthing classes three years ago. Looking out the window as the pain finally ceased, she hoped nothing, like a moose, would delay them from getting to the hospital. She wanted no surprises.

What felt like ages later, Andrew finally dropped Jennifer off at the doors to the hospital and went in search of a parking space. It should have been simple, considering it was around 8:30 p.m.; after-hours were prime parking time with so many coveted spots available. Slamming her door and wincing at the noise that broke the stillness, Jennifer took a steadying breath.

At first, she foolishly tried the main doors. Locked. *Right. It's after hours*, she thought. She headed to the emergency entrance, and after a slight pause to lean against the building and sway, thanks to a contraction, she finally made it to an open door. Entering under the fluorescent glare, she shuffled to the emergency reception. The waiting room had a few people scattered about, sitting in utter boredom for their name to be called. Luckily, Jennifer only needed to register. Then, she was supposed to head straight upstairs to the maternity ward. Hopefully, the doctor was in.

So began the administrative process; information was sought and given for verification: name, date of birth, current address. Somewhere after her name but before her address, another contraction struck. Clutching the counter and swaying her hips, Jennifer breathed in quick breaths. As soon as it was over, she looked up with a grimace on her face.

"I feel like I need to push," breathed Jennifer. The room was silent, the occasional murmurs she'd heard moments before halting abruptly.

The emergency room clerk stared back, eyes wide and mouth slightly parted. The hum of the vending machine provided a steady drone. Somebody coughed. Looking around briefly, as if searching for the answer or divine intervention, the clerk reached over and lifted the receiver of the phone. After a brief pause, she began muttering quickly to the other side. Andrew finally returned, touching Jennifer's back in a brief caress before immediately departing in search of a wheelchair. He returned to the desk moments later, but Jennifer was long gone. He looked around frantically, gripping the handles of the wheelchair tightly. Without missing a beat, every head in the waiting room lifted a hand and pointed toward the elevator. Andrew quickly followed their direction.

It felt like she was sitting on a ball. This was happening too fast! Jennifer had been pacing the elevator like a caged animal, waiting for Andrew to arrive, putting her arm through the door every time it started to close. She wanted a comfortable birth, not one in this elevator, thank you very much! Thankfully, he made it before she had to decide. "I'm not that big!" said Jennifer sharply when he came around the corner, pushing his prize. It was double-wide, a black behemoth. Jennifer eyed it with distaste. But having waddled through the hospital in discomfort this far, Jennifer knew she wouldn't make it upstairs without it. With a grimace, she eased herself down. *You could fit two of me on this thing*, she thought to herself.

The doors closed unencumbered.

Arriving on the fourth floor, Andrew wheeled a huffing and puffing Jennifer to the nurses' station. There was barely a moment between the contractions now. Just as the crescendo was departing, another would leap up in its wake. The nurse immediately rose from inside her fortress. She attempted to ask Jennifer questions, but Jennifer was too far gone, unable to get a word or two out before another contraction would knock her down, sweeping away the rest of her words.

"Straight to the case room!" the nurse declared, pivoting herself out from behind her desk and setting off briskly down the hallway.

Rolling along like a whirlwind of motion, they passed rooms both empty and occupied. In most of the rooms, sweet, sleeping babies were cradled by their exhausted mothers. Heads turned and watched the trio's progress until they went through the double doors down to the birthing wing. They swept through the case room door. Finally, they were where they were meant to be. Jennifer was afraid to stand. If she stood now, she was afraid the baby would fall out. No passing go, no collecting $200! Andrew must have sensed her dilemma. Taking her by both hands, he pulled her up to stand. But it was too late – sploosh! Everything let go like a geyser, amniotic fluid splashing all over the black behemoth wheelchair. This wasn't how Jennifer expected it to go. Where were the hours walking the corridors? It wasn't nearly this fast with her first. This time was so different. Jennifer's mind was swimming.

Finally ensconced on the hospital bed, time slowed for a brief moment. The partner to the nurse was still MIA; the doctor had yet to show his face. They wished they were home, comfortable in their own bed. The second nurse finally arrived at a run; she had been busy with another patient. Everything resumed its blur of motion and information. The cervix was checked. The head was right there! This baby didn't want to wait for anybody.

The new nurse came up beside Jennifer with the fetal monitor while the first nurse puttered, getting things ready for when the doctor arrived. Squirting the cold gel onto Jennifer's belly, she started moving the monitor around to check on the baby, pushing the fetal monitor all around. Only static sounded in the room.

But there was no heartbeat.

The nurses shared a glance. It should have been easy to find the heartbeat of a term baby. It should have been galloping along, ready to meet the world. The silence beared down, suffocating in its implications.

With a determined gleam in her eye, the first nurse, the one who greeted us so readily, donned some gloves and gave a nod. This baby had to come *now*. There was no time to wait for the doctor to arrive. Jennifer was relieved to finally be allowed to push. It almost felt good.

The head popped out easily. So much hair! Then Jennifer was told not to push. The umbilical cord was wrapped around the baby's neck and was too short to fit around its head. Lifting the cord as much as she safely could, the nurse handed Andrew the scissors first, giving him a gentle nudge, and he cut the cord.

Like a little fish swimming in the water, the rest of the baby flowed out. *She was out*. A girl! The euphoria was short-lived, though. There was no cry to herald the new life. No balling fists in birthing fury. She was laying limp in the nurse's hands, suspended in a moment that would be burned forever into Jennifer's mind. Those tiny toes and little fingers, suspended in midair. Everyone, hyper-focused on the tiny being, the lifeless body.

The ticking of the clock sounded louder and louder in Jennifer's ears. Tick. Tock.

The nurse glided across the room to the warming bed, placing the lifeless bundle down. No one dared breathe.

The first nurse, so in control from the moment she was accosted by a frantic pair of soon-to-be parents, lifted the receiver attached to the wall, intending to call a "Code Pink." The silence cut through the air. Jennifer knew something was wrong, but no one would come out and say it. Where was the cry? It felt as if everyone in the room stopped breathing along with her baby. The air became stale, the room was silent, the light was too bright.

Then, a tiny cough broke through the air. Then, a piercing cry shattered the silence. All eyes were upon the little bundle whose voice was now wailing.

The little bundle, tiny and pink, was placed in Jennifer's arms at long last. A feeling of peacefulness flooded her. The nurses began puttering as the new family was acquainted. This night could have ended so differently. Thank God it did not.

Suddenly, the door to the room swung open and a man rushed in, abruptly interrupting the calm. The doctor surveyed the scene.

"I guess I owe the nurses another pizza," he said casually. Nobody spoke, as if in disbelief. With a grin, Jennifer gazed at her sleeping babe. The doctor wasn't needed after all.

About Jennifer

Jennifer Osmond, from Badger, Newfoundland, currently lives in Clarenville, Newfoundland, where she is raising her three beautiful daughters with her husband of nearly 12 years. When she learned about a writing contest involving birth stories, she knew exactly what story she could contribute. The pregnancy with her second child highlights the challenges of smalltown hospitals, where there are only a handful of OB/GYNs on staff. After hours is a whole other ballgame to be won.

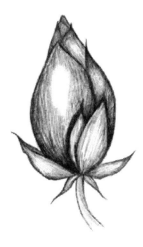

Throughout most of history, until about a hundred years ago, almost all women gave birth at home, surrounded by midwife, friends, and family. In England, these helpers were assembled by the father, after knocking door to door, or 'nidgeting,' throughout the village. In sixteenth century France, that task of locating the sage-femme was simpler because there would have been a sign with symbols, such as a woman holding a baby, or a cradle marked with a fleur-de-lis, handing outside her house. Once in attendance, these women would assist not just in the birth, but in taking care of mother and baby postpartum, from dressing the infant to changing the bed linens, to feeding the husband, knowing that such favors would be returned.

—**Tina Cassidy,** *The Surprising History of How We Are Born*

At Light Speed

by Lisa Brenner
Kitchener, Ontario

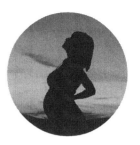

During my first pregnancy, I learned all that I could about natural pregnancy, birth, and baby care, and I planned on having a water birth. After only a short time being in the birth pool, my midwife asked me to get out of the pool so she could check dilation. I was told I was fully dilated, and as another contraction came on, I had felt like I wasn't able to move, and I ended up giving birth on my back on my bed.

With my second pregnancy, I was hoping to give birth in a more upright position. I had thought that being on all fours would be the most comfortable for me. As my waters naturally broke, we discovered the presence of thick meconium, and I was told I needed to transfer to the hospital, and ultimately, birthed my baby while on my back again.

So, when I discovered I was pregnant for a third time, I was determined to give birth in a more favourable position for both myself and my baby.

Three days before my due date, I had an appointment with an OB/GYN. My plan was to have a home birth with midwives, but due to my "advanced maternal age" (I was a month shy of 41 years old and had already had two uneventful pregnancies, and easy, relatively quick births), I was required to see an OB/GYN in case I needed to be induced, as it wasn't recommended that I go past my due date. Thank goodness it didn't come to that!

My appointment was scheduled for 9:10 a.m. I woke up around 8:30 a.m. and thought that I should eat something before I left for the clinic, but for some reason, the thought of food didn't appeal to me. As I waited for my partner, Premdas, to get ready, I noticed that I was feeling a bit off – a little bit achy, but nothing major.

When we arrived at our doctor's office, we were told that we'd have to wait, as she had been at a birth earlier that morning and had not yet arrived at the clinic.

As we took a seat in the waiting area, the discomfort I had experienced earlier returned, but this time, it felt much stronger, like a contraction. The feeling kept increasing, coming in waves, and getting closer and closer together.

Finally, the nurse called me to the back. I sat down as she started asking questions, and after one look at me, she said, "You're in labour!" All I could say was "Yes." I was surprised, as I really didn't think I was exhibiting any signs. In fact, I think I was still in denial that it was happening. She asked me if I'd be okay to go back out and sit in the waiting room, assuring me that the doctor would be with me shortly.

Back in the waiting room, which was near capacity at this point, the contractions continued to gain momentum. I focused on my breathing while I squeezed Premdas' hand. I felt self-conscious and a bit nervous. I should have been home. Thankfully, it wasn't long before I was taken to a room to wait for the doctor.

A few minutes later, the doctor quickly breezed into the room, sat down, and whirled around to look at me, exclaiming, "You're in labour!" I found it quite funny to hear this exact statement twice. I guess when you spend a lot of time around birthers, you know just by looking at them when they're in labour.

She performed a quick cervical check and said that I was about 6 cm dilated and around 80% effaced. "You're going to have your baby today!" she said excitedly. Then, she asked, "What would you like to do? Go home and have your home birth?" to which I replied, "Yes!"

She paged the midwife, Minke, who immediately called back. The doctor filled her in on what was happening, said that I was doing great, and that I was going to go back home to have my home birth. Minke said she'd meet us at our house.

As we left the doctor's office to make our way back to the car, I kept pausing to breathe through the contractions. I stopped walking to lean on my partner several times: in the hallway, in the elevator, on the steps outside the building, on the way to the parking lot, and once more before stepping into the car.

It was only a five-minute drive from home. Not a word passed between Premdas and me as I gripped the door handle and focused my energy on my breath. A brief moment of panic passed through my thoughts as my "thinking brain" kicked in, realizing what was about to happen once again. I pushed the thoughts aside as I relaxed into the present moment, trusting that my body and breath knew just what to do.

Once parked in the driveway, Premdas helped me out of the car as another strong contraction came on. I had to lean on the wall of the house for support. When it passed, he asked if I needed a minute. All I could do was shake my head and move quickly up the path and into the house. In my mind, I knew I needed to get inside before I hit the transition phase, as I would no longer be able to move. I was determined not to have this baby in my driveway.

Another wave hit before I could even remove my shoes. When it passed, I went straight into my bedroom and felt another contraction coming on. I struggled to remove my clothing, as I knew it wouldn't be long before the baby's arrival.

I remained standing while holding on to the change table for support, when the next contraction brought out a deep, long, moaning exhale.

Transition!

Now I could only take quick, sharp inhales that extended into deep and low, long, groaning exhales. Out of nowhere, I heard Minke's voice saying, "Lisa, you're doing great!"

With my back turned to the door, I heard Minke call out to Premdas, instructing him to go to her car to get the emergency birthing kit. A moment later, I heard it hit the floor behind me as she unrolled it. Minke must have known by the sounds that I was making that my baby's birth was imminent, because as she was struggling to open the suitcase of supplies, she said to go ahead and push if I felt the urge to with the next contraction. As I gently bore down, my water broke with a loud pop and startled me as it splashed everywhere. Minke reassured me that it was just the waters breaking and that the fluid was clear, so not to worry.

The next contraction came, and I felt my baby's body descending. With one more gentle push, I birthed my beautiful little boy. Later, my partner would say that it looked like our son came out at the speed of light.

His birth happened so quickly that his cord snapped with a popping sound. Minke caught him and handed him to my partner as she clamped the baby's cord. Later, when inspecting the placenta, she mentioned that the cord was quite short.

Minke assisted me from standing to lying down on my bed as the second midwife, Cheryl, came through the door. Once settled, Premdas kneeled beside me and leaned in to kiss me as he gently rolled the baby from his chest to mine.

It all happened so incredibly fast. Minke was only present for 11 minutes before my son, Arjuna, was born. He arrived at 11:06 a.m., which was just under two hours from my scheduled appointment that morning, and the first inkling of a contraction.

About Lisa

Lisa lives in Kitchener, Ontario with her partner and three children. She is an Ayurvedic practitioner, a pre/postnatal yoga teacher, Reiki master, and doula. She weaves all of these beautiful practices together to provide loving care for birthers and their sweet babes. The immediate postpartum period has her heart. You can connect with her on all social networks as Wise Roots Therapies.

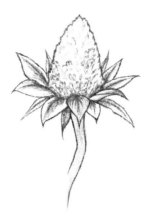

Drugs aside, many in myth and reality have sworn they would give up anything to avoid the agony of childbirth. Even sex. The Greek goddess Artemis was so terrified by her mother's suffering at her own birth that she asked Zeus for the favor of eternal virginity. She changed her mind, though, seduced by Endymion, and ended up giving birth to fifty daughters.

—**Tina Cassidy**, *Birth: The Surprising History of How We Are Born*

Miles to Journey Through

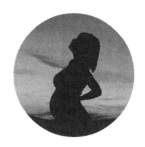

by Aly Guildford
Muskoka, Ontario

"If you don't score an 8/8 during your ultrasound, you will need to be induced," my midwife informed me over the phone. I was 10 days overdue at the time.

This was my first baby, and even though I knew most first-time moms go over their due date, I always thought labour would start on its own. So, at 9:45 a.m. on October 17th, which also happened to be my birthday, we drove 21 km to the hospital for the ultrasound – an ultrasound that I was supposed to have had on the Friday before, but the hospital never informed me of my appointment.

Twenty minutes later, my partner and I are told to wait for the results. Turns out, I did not score an 8/8. My amniotic fluid was low, and I needed to be induced. My midwife and the on-call doctor were called to meet me upstairs.

First, my midwife did a vaginal exam. Then the on-call doctor examined me as well, although I had never met them before. My birth plan consisted of maintaining my modesty and only having one midwife examine me vaginally, but sometimes, plans are thrown out the window.

I was treated to a stretch-and-sweep, and Cervidil to trigger contractions. We were instructed to come back at 9 p.m. to have it taken out.

Finally, at 1 p.m., we left the hospital and emerged into the pouring rain. To save some money, we chose not to park in the hospital parking lot, but we didn't expect it to rain. Laughing, we quickly walked down two hills to our car and drove back to our apartment.

Because it was my 21st birthday, we had invited our families over to celebrate. We enjoyed the company, the cake, the presents, and especially the excitement over possibly welcoming our son into the world on the very same day. How cool would that be? I remember sitting there with everyone trying to join the conversation, but I was so focused on rubbing my belly and moving side to side to dull the aches that were beginning.

Once everyone left, around 9 p.m., we drove back to the hospital. The midwife and the on-call doctor took out the Cervidil and, to my surprise, came some of my mucus plug with it. They confirmed my cervix was soft and I was most likely experiencing contractions, and so, we returned home to rest and wait for labour to begin.

At 1 a.m. on October 18th (yep, no baby on my birthday), the pain was getting stronger. I tried a hot pack, a hot bath, walking, resting, all while my partner binged on Skittles. Finally, we called my mom to bring over some Tylenol. We also called our midwife over, as we had been timing my contractions for an hour and they were one minute long and a couple minutes apart. When she arrived, she checked for dilation. I was 5 cm dilated and she said I could be admitted into the hospital.

I nodded vigorously, and my mom said she would meet us back at the hospital later in the morning.

It was 3 a.m. by the time we arrived at the hospital. I soaked in the soothing labouring tub while my partner had a nap.

According to my midwife, I had an abnormal contraction cycle because she couldn't see them properly on the monitors. I had to tell her when they were happening, although it was hard to say when one ended or began sometimes.

The pain kept getting stronger, so I used the TENS machine to abate it, but the contractions continued to get stronger, longer, and more frequent.

I tried the laughing gas, but it didn't do anything for me. I had a vaginal exam again; I was 7 cm dilated.

We decided to break my water to further induce me.

By 11 a.m., I was extremely fed up with the pain and lack of rest, so I asked for any type of medication other than epidural. I was also starting to get worried as it was becoming more difficult to hear the baby's heartbeat. I thought some pain medication might help me to calm down and rest so that maybe we could see how the baby was doing. As my midwife was preparing the medication, I curled on my side, squeezed my eyes shut, and groaned, "Why does it feel like my uterus is pushing?"

She turned around, shocked, her mouth agape. She dropped the needle and coaxed me into turning over for another vaginal check. Sure enough, I was ready to go, fully dilated. She rushed over to her phone, called the second midwife, and rushed back to me.

"Alright, you need to bear down with the pushing feeling," she instructed me, settling herself between my legs. My partner had to go outside at that point because my grandma and his mother decided to pay us a visit. My modesty was honestly the last thing I was thinking about; I was in full birthing mode. I wasn't thinking about anything, only aware of what my body was telling me to do. I knew this was it, and…

I was ready.

I kept my eyes closed and my hands were gripping the bed rails. Once I began pushing, it felt so good, until his head was crowning. My midwife had to run and call the nurses. I felt the ring of fire as his head came through, and my partner told me he could see it.

I thought pushing would take longer, but my midwife rushed back, accompanied by two nurses who placed themselves on either side of me supporting my legs with knees up to my chest to help get my baby's shoulders out. They all kept chanting, "You're doing amazing," and I truly felt amazing. I was this strong, capable woman, bearing a child naturally, as I planned.

At 11:41 a.m., October 18th, my baby boy, Oliver Miles, was born and he was immediately placed onto my chest. He was 9 lbs, 3 oz, and 21 inches long, with the most perfectly round-shaped head. He wasn't crying, but his eyes were open. It was such a beautiful and shocking sight to see my newborn son looking up at me. As soon as I held my baby, I forgot all about the pain, basking in his first moments. I felt nothing else.

After my partner had cut the cord, the nurses said goodbye, a midwife took my son to be cleaned up, and my other midwife instructed me to help her guide the placenta out. I pushed and a gush of blood came out, then I pushed again, and the placenta swiftly slid out. Only, I kept on bleeding. Suddenly, everything happened fast. My midwife barked out an order and the student midwife came at me with a large syringe. She gripped my knee, and I blurted out, "Will it hurt?" She answered yes and stuck it in my thigh with no warning. It definitely hurt but I later learned it was full of oxytocin to help my bleeding to slow.

After I had some time to rest, I was told I could get up and have a shower. I swung my legs over the bed and walked to the shower with my midwife. As I was waiting for the water to get warm, I said, "I need to sit down." The next thing I knew, I was laying on the ground with my head in my student midwife's lap and the other trying to rouse me awake – I had fainted from loss of blood. I looked at my partner, who was holding the baby and I realized I couldn't hear anything, nor could I feel my legs. It took a few moments for all my senses to come back. I was told not to move and had to drink ginger ale to perk myself up.

I sat to shower while the midwives monitored just outside the bathroom. The water falling onto my back was the most incredible feeling on my worn-out body, the warmth of it carrying away the chill and shakes I had after giving birth. Once I was showered, my midwife helped me into a huge pair of padded underwear, and we were moved to another room so I could stay overnight.

Oliver's middle name, Miles, continues to be a testament to our journey as a family, even four years later. We experienced a lot of struggles through postpartum, breastfeeding, solids, and development but we have come so far from the newborn who wouldn't latch, to the infant who wouldn't sleep, to the toddler who couldn't speak.

Birthing my baby naturally made me feel invincible, and I was proud to have followed in the footsteps of my grandmother and my mother.

About Aly

Aly has settled in Huntsville Ontario. She met her husband in high school and they have been together ever since. They currently have two children, a son born in 2016 and a daughter born in 2019. Aly is a registered early childhood educator and uses her knowledge on a daily basis. She enjoys reading and writing, and so she was thrilled to contribute a meaningful story about such a precious event. Midwives attended both her births and their support was out of this world. She believes everyone could benefit from having a midwife and/or a doula.

Birth Sharing Circles: Hosting Your Own

Literary Birth Sharing Circles

Following each annual Birth Story Writing Contest, the Doula Support Foundation hosted a different kind of reading event, which we called a Birth Sharing Circle. Sharing circles are a core part of many Indigenous cultures, including in North America. We are grateful to Indigenous communities for the wisdom and expertise they hold around this practice, and from which we borrow. For us, our Birthing Sharing Circles allowed those who assessed the stories (the jurors and readers) and those who wrote the stories to meet and share their experiences of participating in the contest. For the writers, it gave them the opportunity to reflect on the process of writing and sharing their birth stories. We also made these circles open to expectant parents and birth health providers who wanted to join and listen.

Our Birth Sharing Circles were grounded in compassion and centred on listening to and celebrating those who shared their birth stories. That is, as in the Indigenous tradition of sharing circles, listeners are encouraged to intentionally open their ears and hearts to the stories being shared from a place of connection and care. This format created an incredibly powerful experience for all who attended and left us all with a deep sense of solidarity and awe for those who birth.

The first Birth Sharing Circle was in person and not recorded. With the onset of the global COVID-19 pandemic, our Birth Sharing Circles in 2020 and 2021 had to be on Zoom. They can be viewed at www.doulasupport.org/book-page. We were worried about losing the sense of magic and connection through doing the Circle on Zoom, but the events did not disappoint!

Community Birth Sharing Circles

Inspired by these Birth Sharing Circles, the Doula Support Foundation subsequently organized a few Community Birth Sharing Circles. These were intended to provide a space for healing and empowerment, and were all, once again, incredibly powerful, despite being held virtually.

The goal of this book is to promote a more positive and empowering culture around birth; to this end, we want to provide some guidelines for holding a Birth Sharing Circle for those who wish to do so. Our hope is that people will organize their own Birth Sharing Circles amongst peer groups and local communities, across Canada and beyond.

Guidelines for Holding a Community Birth Sharing Circle

A Birth Sharing Circle is an occasion for all participants to be heard, respected, and valued. The space should be open to all birthing parents, new, young and old, whether they want to share or listen. The most important element is the deep listening, which means that participants withhold judgement, comments, and advice. The circle should be designed around offering a safe environment for birthgivers to speak freely from their heart, and an invitation for others to listen and hold space for those who wish to share.

The circle can follow this rough outline:

- ♦ Opening discussion from the facilitator.
- ♦ Grounding exercise (e.g., short group breathing and meditation exercise).
- ♦ Prompts and reflection.
- ♦ A round of brief introductions.
- ♦ Sharing stories (about 5-10 minutes per person, depending on how many participants are present).

- Closing the circle.
- Announcements, if any.
- Sharing of food and beverage.

Guidelines for an Empowering and Powerful Circle:

1. Plan for circles to last 1.5-2 hours. If in person, organize seats/space for everyone to sit in a circle. Choose an object from nature (e.g., feather, rock, stick) that can be held by the person sharing and pass it to the next person once she has finished sharing.

2. Creating a safe place. All that is said in the circle stays anonymous outside. If one feels they want to share something fruitful outside the circle, names and other identifying information must be left out.

3. Each participant respects a limited time to share, so all have time to do so. It is helpful to ask those with multiple birth experiences to choose one to focus on. The facilitator can use a sign or bell to remind people that two minutes is left for her/him to share.

4. Practicing deep listening and giving each participant our full attention. That means acting as her witness and supporting without interruption or asking questions. Stepping out of judgement especially if triggered, remaining present during the circle, and refraining from the practice of listening to respond. Instead, listen to learn and be curious.

5. When you are the person speaking, trust that whatever comes to mind and heart to share is exactly what you need to share. We release ourselves from expectations or any script.

6. Sharing our personal experience rather than "teaching" our ideas or philosophies or asking participation from the others such as signing, breathing exercises, etc.

7. Have a short break halfway through.

8. Brief time at the end for any relevant community announcements after the circle has been closed.

9. Those who have little ones who can nurse/nap/stay in one's lap are welcome to join.

10. Decide if you want to have a potluck or some beverage to share after the circle.

Essential Evidence-Based Guidance for Birth

You've simmered in, contemplated, and reflected on so many beautifully written birth stories from different voices across a range of experiences. Through reading these stories, you have *felt* what birth can be like. You know that birth can be as wildly unpredictable as it can be transformative. Nevertheless, there are key ingredients for creating the conditions for a positive birth experience where birthgivers feel cared for, respected, and heard. There are also deeply rooted inequalities that make realizing this goal more challenging for some birthgivers, and it's valuable for us to understand these systemic barriers so that we can change them, and support those experiencing them better and with more compassion. Bringing together the voices of a variety of practitioners, clinicians, and scholars in birth and perinatal care, this section of the book covers essential evidence-based guidance for creating the conditions for positive and empowering birth experiences for all.

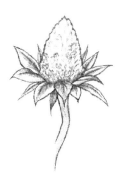

What is a Doula and How Can They Help Me?

by Laura Pascoe

> *If a doula were a drug, it would be unethical not to use it.*
> —Dr. John Kennell, pioneering doula researcher and pediatrician

What is a Doula?

Doulas are trained companions rooted in ancient traditions. The term "doula" is translated from Greek to mean "a woman who serves" (Dukehart, 2011). In the context of childbirth, birth doulas are trained to provide emotional, physical, informational, and advocacy support during pregnancy, throughout labour and birth, and in the initial weeks postpartum. If a birthing person has a partner or other loved one, doulas also provide invaluable support to the partner, many of whom have never themselves attended a birth, and doulas provide guidance and essential skills to partners so they can best support their loved one.

Birth doulas support clients alongside any healthcare provider (e.g., midwife, obstetrician, family doctor) and in any location, including home, birth centres, and hospitals—although doulas were excluded from some hospitals in the initial phases of the COVID-19 global pandemic. Doulas are usually hired by the birthing person, with some labour and delivery wards offering onsite doulas who are either paid or volunteer. A doula's primary responsibility and role are connected to the needs and wellbeing of the birthing person—not to a midwife, obstetrician, nurse, or even baby (Dekker, 2019). In this way, birth doulas provide focused and continuous support to the birthing person to ensure they feel supported, respected, and heard. Clinical tasks, such as taking blood pressure, monitoring the baby, or catching (delivering) the baby are not in a doula's scope of work.

Doulas also do not make decisions for their clients. However, the question of if, how, and in what circumstances it is appropriate for a doula to advocate on behalf of their client (as opposed to making decisions for them) has been increasingly debated in and outside of the doula community. Historically, many doula training organizations actively discouraged doulas from engaging in advocacy, citing concern that doulas might lose favour of healthcare providers or be refused entry to hospitals. Yet, there has been a growing call for doulas to identify advocacy as a key part of their role, in line with their primary responsibility to the birthing person. This has also been in the context of increased visibility of biases and discrimination that contribute to racial disparities in maternal health and birth outcomes, obstetric violence, and the ways that the medicalization of childbirth often deprioritizes the needs and preferences of birthing people.

Rebecca Dekker, founder of the Evidence-Based Birth website and repository of evidence-based birthing information, defines advocacy in the context of childbirth as "supporting the birthing person in their right to make decisions about their own body and baby" (Dekker, 2019). For example, if a healthcare provider enters a labouring woman's hospital room and tells her it is time for a cervical exam, and her doula knows that a) a cervical exam should always be a choice; b) their client wants minimal cervical exams; and c) their client is focused on her contractions and is unable to speak for herself, then a doula might say something like, "Thank you for checking on her! She mentioned wanting to minimize the number of vaginal exams. When this contraction is finished let's see how she is feeling. Thank you so much again for providing such good care." In this way, the doula is ensuring the client's preferences are respected while freeing her client to focus on labour, and does so in a way that is kind and respectful to the healthcare provider. See the advocacy section below for more examples of what doula advocacy support might look like.

The doula profession is female-dominated, but there are also many doulas who do not identify as women, including less common male doulas (Dorward, 2018; Vargas, 2021). Encouragingly, there is also a growing number of Black, Brown, and Indigenous doulas offering services, although more are needed to ensure that all birthing people have access to doulas who resonate with and meet their needs. A sustainable funding model is needed to support Indigenous doula services in Canada (Wodtke et al., 2022), and financial assistance to reduce barriers for Black and Brown doulas to obtain training is also needed (Paynter et al., 2022). All families can benefit from a doula, and we (at the Doula Support Foundation) strongly believe that every birthing person who wants a doula deserves to have one.

Doulas for All Your Reproductive Needs

In addition to birth doulas, there are also doulas trained for other areas of one's reproductive journey, from abortion to fertility/infertility to pregnancy loss and postpartum. Abortion doulas, also sometimes called full-spectrum doulas, provide support in cases of pregnancy termination, including answering questions about what to expect, attending appointments as needed, and providing physical and emotional support during the abortion process, including at home in cases of medical abortion. Pregnancy loss doulas are trained to provide support in cases of expected or unexpected pregnancy loss, such as in cases of termination as well as miscarriage and stillbirth. Pregnancy loss doulas can be particularly valuable for grieving parents navigating an overwhelming set of decisions and emotions while in shock and/or mourning.

Fertility doulas support parents along their journey to pregnancy and parenthood, including informational support to navigate the fertility process, as well as emotional and physical support to ease anxiety, cope with challenges, and promote wellbeing. Postpartum doulas provide support specific to the postpartum period and up to a year after the baby's birth. This can include feeding and sleep support, overnight care, cooking meals, light housekeeping, and emotional support related to birth and adjusting to parenthood/adding a child to the family. Some doulas specialize in particular areas, such as birth, fertility, or postpartum, while others are trained across multiple areas and can support a client across their journey (for example, through a birth and postpartum period, which is then followed by a need for abortion doula support, or through years of infertility and then throughout a successful pregnancy, birth, and into postpartum). As this book focused on birth stories, the following section on evidence about doulas focuses on birth doula support.

What Does the Evidence Say About Doulas?

Available evidence on birth doula care continues to confirm the valuable support doulas provide. For one, birthing people actually feel less pain when a doula is present (Dekker, 2019). A 2017 systematic review (which is a rigorous process of synthesizing and assessing research in order to facilitate evidence-based decision-making) analyzed research from randomized controlled trials covering nearly 16,000 birthgivers, and found that continuous support in childbirth is beneficial, particularly when that person is a doula (National Partnership for Women & Families, 2018). In short, research shows that doula support improves birth outcomes, supports the birthing person in having their needs met and preferences respected, and increases the likelihood of having a positive birth experience. Specifically, researchers found that having a doula (National Partnership for Women & Families, 2018):

- Reduced the likelihood of having a negative birth experience by 35%.
- Reduced the likelihood of experiencing an unnecessary caesarean birth.
- Increased the likelihood of having a spontaneous vaginal birth by at least 15%.
- Reduced the use of synthetic oxytocin.
- Decreased the need for pain medication.
- Decreased the likelihood of the newborn being admitted to the special/intensive care nursery.

Other research has found that doula support leads to improved bonding between parents and their baby, increases the likelihood of successfully initiating breast/chestfeeding, and reduces risk factors for postpartum depression (Dekker, 2019; Dukehart, 2011; Gruber et al., 2013).

What Does Birth Doula Support Look Like in Practice?

To help make clear what doula support looks like in real time, the following section provides an overview doula support in practice, based on the five pillars of support (emotional, physical, informational, partner, and advocacy):

Emotional

- Reassurance.

- Encouragement and praise.

- Soothing presence.

- Validation and processing for the birthing person's worries, fears, and experiences (e.g., making space for emotions beyond "healthy mom, healthy baby").

- Continuous presence that is attuned to the birthing person's needs and preferences.

- Keeping them company.

Physical

- Massage.

- Relaxation techniques, including breathing and body relaxation techniques.

- Reminders to and assistance in movement and positioning that can speed up labour and/or ease discomfort/pain.

- Creating an environment that mirrors the birthing person's state and preferences (e.g., dimming lights, upbeat or calm music, candles).

- Offering sips of water between contractions and sustenance when needed/desired.

- Breast/chestfeeding support after birth

Informational

- Helping to prepare the pregnant person (and partner) on what to expect during labour, birth, and postpartum.

- Help in finding evidence-based information to guide preparation and decision-making.

- Guidance throughout labour and birth, such as support in identifying the onset of active labour.

- Suggestions for and guidance in utilizing calming, coping, and non-medical pain management techniques for labour and birth, as well as movement and positions to try.

- Guidance on birth preference plan, if desired.

- Logistical support, such as a checklist for what to pack on one's hospital bag.

- Help with identifying a support system and with planning for the postpartum period.

Partner

- Teaching the partner how to use pain management techniques for the labouring person.

- Providing them a space to ask questions and/or process their experiences of supporting labour and witnessing birth in the early postpartum period.

- Reassurance and encouragement for their role (e.g., "I know she looks like she's in a lot of pain, but she's in transition right now and this is a good thing! Keep encouraging her that she can do it").

Advocacy

The following are taken from the Evidence-Based Birth website (Dekker, 2019):

- Encouraging the birthing person or their partner to ask questions and verbalize their preferences.

- Asking the birthing person what they want.

- Supporting the birthing person's decision.

- Amplifying the mother's voice if she is being dismissed, ignored, or not heard (e.g., "Excuse me, she's trying to tell you something. I wasn't sure if you heard her or not").

- Creating space and time for the birthing family so that they can ask questions, gather evidence-based information, and make decisions without feeling pressured.

- Facilitating communication between the parents and their healthcare providers.

- Teaching the birthing person and partner positive communication techniques.

- If a birthing person is not aware that a provider is about to perform an intervention, the doula could point out what it appears the nurse or physician is about to do, and ask the birthing person if they have any questions about what is about to happen. For example, if it looks like the provider is about to perform an episiotomy without the person's consent: "Dr. Smith has scissors in his hand. Do you have any questions about what he is wanting to do with the scissors?"

Choosing a Healthcare Provider and the Birth Setting

by Laura Pascoe and Josée Leduc

She stood, bent over the bed, moaning softly to herself as she swayed, back and forth, back and forth, back and forth. She'd been at this for hours, and the intensity kept growing, but she knew she could keep going, at least for the next contraction. And maybe the next. All she knew was that her team was around her, and she trusted them to support her.

Putting thought into the choices of birth setting and healthcare provider is important in pregnancy. These factors can greatly influence how labour and delivery unfolds and how one feels about the experience.

We have included this section to help support birthgivers in being informed and prepared, including by taking "an active role in selecting their caregiver or birth setting in early pregnancy" (Jimenez et al., 2010). The model of care provided varies significantly among healthcare providers, as do policies and protocols from hospital to hospital. Understanding these factors alongside your own preferences and rights is key to setting yourself up for a positive birth experience.

Humans are heavily influenced by both the people and the environment that surround them, and birth is a moment where these factors can be particularly impactful. In most provinces in Canada, birthgivers have three maternity care provider options: midwife, family physician, or obstetrician, with their comprehensive pregnancy and birth care covered by provincial healthcare (Public Health Agency of Canada, 2020). However, this is not true in all provinces and all communities. For one, many Indigenous birthgivers living in rural areas or on remote reserves must contend with the One Health Canada evacuation policy, which requires them to be taken away from their communities to birth in urban hospitals, leaving them no choice regarding their healthcare providers (Lawford et al., 2018) and birth setting. However, the Inuit in the Nunavik region of northern Quebec have "re-matriated" birth by bringing it back into their communities. This process started in the town of Puvirnituq, where a profession homebirth midwife, Jennifer Stonier, was brought in to train Indigenous women to become professional midwives, who work in a maternity centre that is 2-8 hours away by plane from the nearest hospital. This model has worked so well that it has spread throughout the entire Nunavik region.

Today, childbearers get the majority of their prenatal care from obstetricians (58%), family physicians (34%), and midwives (6%) (Public Health Agency of Canada, 2020). This is in contrast to many other industrialized countries, such as New Zealand, the Netherlands, and Japan, where midwives are responsible for the majority of maternity care. While the proportion of births in Canada that obstetricians attend has remained relatively stable since the beginning of the 21st century, family physicians are providing fewer people prenatal care and attending fewer births than in the past, while the midwifery workforce is slowly but steadily growing (see below).

Things to Consider in Choosing a Provider

All maternity care providers have at least two patients to attend to: the pregnant/postpartum person and the baby/babies. All maternity healthcare providers are highly trained and certified. Nevertheless, they have different training and varying perspectives that they bring to birth (even within the same profession). It is helpful to know and understand how maternity care providers trained in different professions view birth (and their role in facilitating birth) to better inform one's choice of care provider.

Midwifery

Midwifery has been around as long as birth. For millennia across the world over, childbirth was perceived as the domain of women and midwifery was, traditionally and still largely is, a female-dominated profession (in every country, only around one percent of midwives are men). Historically, midwives were trained by other midwives and gained extensive knowledge and expertise in birth, herbal remedies, and other medical services, and were highly respected members of their communities.

Midwives have been practicing in Canada for centuries. Indigenous midwives in Canada provided essential and highly skilled services in their communities before white settlers outlawed their practices, which compromised access to quality maternity care for generations of Indigenous birthgivers. In the broader Canadian context, the growing interest in controlling and managing the domain of birth by medical institutions and their (male) physicians came with efforts to undermine and eventually outlaw the midwifery profession. It was only in the 1990s, at the demand of Canadian birthgivers desiring greater ownership over their birthing process and experience, that midwifery returned from the fringes and once again become a well-respected and regulated profession in Canada. In 2019, professional midwives only attended around 11% of Canadian births, yet that percentage is much higher in provinces such as Ontario and British Columbia, where midwives attend around 20% of all births (Association of Ontario Midwives, 2022b). However, due to the lack of supportive legislation in many provinces, there are limited options for formal midwifery training in Canada. At the moment, there is a much higher demand for midwives than available supply.

The training of a Canadian midwife consists of a four-year bachelor's degree that is focused on low-risk pregnancies and births and on identifying complicated cases that need to be transferred to obstetric care. Midwives are expected to gain experience attending both home and hospital births as a standard part of their educational requirements. They are fully trained to provide care from early pregnancy through to at least six weeks postpartum for childbearers and their infants. The postpartum care offered by midwives is patient- and family-centred, with regular at-home or clinic visits in the first weeks postpartum. For example, the value of the midwifery model of postpartum services was recognized in the early months of the COVD-19 pandemic in Kingston, Ontario when midwives responded to a demand for such services by providing them to anyone who needed them.

This resulted in the creation of a new clinic run by the local midwives in collaboration with the local hospital that provides "time-sensitive follow up services for parents and newborns after discharge" and is "intended to provide support to families without existing access to time-sensitive care such as those without existing access to midwifery care, who do not have a family physician, or otherwise face barriers to access" (Goulem, 2022).

The midwifery model of care views birth as a normal and physiologic process that does not inherently require technological interventions. Midwives are trained to promote health and wellness by providing education and support, recognizing childbearers as the primary decision-maker in their care, and encouraging informed decision-making through collaboration with their clients (Malott et al., 2012; Simkin et al., 2018). While 25-30% of midwifery clients plan home births, the remaining 70-75% plan to give birth at a hospital or (if an option) in a birth centre with their midwives present (Vedam et al., 2014). Fears and realities relating to the COVID-19 pandemic increased the number of people interested in or opting for home birth in many contexts (where and for whom this was an option), including Canada and the US, with promising data to show good outcomes (Association of Ontario Midwives, 2022c; Cheng et al., 2022; Daviss et al., 2021; MacDorman et al., 2022).

Family Physicians

The medicalization of birth in the 19th century led to family physicians, or general practitioners, increasingly attending births. As generalists in the field of medicine who focus on primary and comprehensive care for individuals and families across the lifespan, family physicians tend to see birth as a normal physiological event. However, some take a more medicalized approach, depending on their training and perspective. For example, favourability towards planned home births is strongly associated with exposure to birth in home settings, which many family physicians do not receive during their training (Vedam et al., 2014). Family physicians often have detailed knowledge of their patients due to their previous interactions related to primary care, which can be desirable for a birthgiver. They are increasingly sharing care with other maternity care providers, offering much of the prenatal care before transferring care to other family physicians, obstetricians, or midwives (Canadian Institute for Health Information, 2004). Intervention rates among family physicians fall somewhere between those of midwives and obstetricians (Public Health Agency of Canada, 2020).

The training of a family doctor who offers maternity care requires a four-year bachelor's degree and a degree from a medical school (four years), followed by a two-year residency. This training is also focused on low-risk pregnancies. One of the advantages of having a family doctor for maternity care is the continuity of care over the years, as they may become the healthcare provider for all of the family members beyond perinatal care.

Obstetrician/Gynecologist

The first obstetrician-gynecologists (OB/GYN) began practicing in Canada in the 19th century. Prior to that, the first key obstetric invention, forceps-assisted delivery, is attributed to two brothers from the Chamberlen family in 16th-century France. The brothers were trained as barber-surgeons but later gained specialization in obstetrics. The Chamberlen family kept the forceps a profitable secret for well over a century, before others began to design and use their own versions of forceps. By the 18th century, medical professionals understood more of the anatomy and physiology of birth, and wanted to train and become experts in this "new" field of medicine. This was also around the time that "lying in" hospitals were founded, furthering the presence of obstetricians attending births.

OB/GYNs gained popularity through their life-saving treatments, medical pain relief options, and other medical advances that are indispensable for some births, such as in cases of obstructed labour and high-risk pregnancies.

The obstetric model of care sees birth through a biomedical lens, meaning that birth is viewed more as a medical event similar to a disease or illness that requires vigilant monitoring, diagnostics, and treatment as part of the overall management of patient health.

The extensive training and expertise of obstetricians is indispensable for high-risk pregnancies and complicated labours, and medical interventions have saved the lives of many birthgivers and babies. However, due to their training and the contexts in which they work, obstetricians tend to have less time to meet with and answer questions with patients prenatally and during labour. Additionally, they are more likely than other maternity care providers to approach conversations with their patients from a place of authority and knowledge, informing the patient what their options are or, often, what their recommended course of action is. This can lead to a birthgiver being unaware of alternative options or understanding they have a choice in all aspects of their care.

The training of an OB/GYN requires a four-year bachelor's degree and a degree from a medical school followed by internship and residency programs that last five to seven years. They serve as the experts in high-risk pregnancies and complicated labours, and receive surgical training, such as caesarean section. Yet they often have little or no expertise in attending normal physiologic births, and end up perpetuating this skewed experience through technologically intervening in births they attend. This tendency to over-intervene in labours and births has led to Canada's current caesarean birth rate of 28%. It also highlights what Melissa Cheyney and Robbie Davis-Floyd (2019, pg. 8) have called the "obstetric paradox": intervene to keep birth safe, thereby causing harm.

Choosing a Birth Setting

There are three possible places one can choose to give birth: at home, in a freestanding birth centre, or in a hospital. However, some of these choices are not available depending on where in Canada you are located.

At Home

Giving birth at home is a safe choice for candidates with low-risk pregnancies. In Canada, it is mainly midwives who offer this option, though some family physicians will attend home births. However, midwives are still not regulated in Yukon and Prince Edward Island, nor are they accessible in all communities, meaning that not all Canadians have this choice of care available to them. Also, where midwives are practicing, they are in high demand and there is often a long waitlist, which has been compounded by the increased demand for avoiding hospital settings due to risks associated with COVID-19. So it is important to contact a midwife or midwifery clinic early in pregnancy for the best chance of accessing their care. Scholar and midwife Eileen Hutton (2016, p. 332) explains:

> In provinces in which midwifery is regulated, and home birth is a part of that regulation, home birth is well-integrated into the healthcare system. This has resulted in perinatal and neonatal outcomes for women planning home birth that are not different from those for women planning hospital births (Hutton, 2016, p. 332).

In other words, home births are as safe as hospital births in Canada for low-risk pregnancies. In a Canadian study (Vedam et al., 2012) regarding the attitudes of healthcare providers towards planned home birth, almost all registered midwives were very positive about home birth as an option, and the majority of obstetricians and family physicians were opposed to or uncomfortable with home birth. It is to be noted that most OB/GYNs and family doctors have never attended a home birth in their training and are often not aware of the safety equipment that midwives have at their disposal. As such, this is not a choice that is usually offered to pregnant people at the doctor's office, even though, again, studies have shown that it is as safe as hospital birth in places where midwifery is integrated with the healthcare system.

The Pros of Home Birth:

- For many, it is an environment where the birthing person feels safe and comfortable, and therefore, can relax, let go, and concentrate on labouring without disturbance.

- Free to move at any time, without continuous electronic monitoring.[1]

- Possibility to have an "aquadural" (being immersed in water) and a water birth.

- Easier to avoid unwanted medical interventions, such as continuous fetal monitoring, IV, vaginal exams, augmentation, or epidural.

- No need to get in a car or taxi while labouring.

- Care provided by known midwife/midwives who provide medical, emotional, and physical support, and who feels comfortable and confident in the outcome of home birth.

- Attending midwives practice a patient-centred care model, which includes informed consent.

- Attending midwives are trained to foresee complications and be ready to transfer to hospital, if need be.

- Midwives do home visits after birth (no need to travel with a newborn to see the care provider).

- Midwives can help with infant feeding and baby care.

- Possibility to add a doula to support team.

---

[1] For evidence-based information about fetal monitoring see https://evidencebasedbirthacademy.com/dashboard-old/pdf-library/

The Cons of Home Birth (which can also be seen as pros)

- Have to transfer to the hospital for medicated pain relief, should the need arise.
- Have to transfer to the hospital in case of complications with the labour and delivery.
- If you do not feel at ease in your home, whether because of physical environment or because of a partner, then a hospital might be your preferred place to birth.
- If you are afraid of labour and birth, or that something will go wrong, then you might feel safest in a hospital.

At a Birth Centre

There are two birth centres, plus one Indigenous midwife-led centre in Ontario, four in Alberta, one in Manitoba, and 21 *maisons de naissance* in Québec.

A birth centre is a place where pregnant people can receive a full range of midwifery services. It provides a large, home-like setting where birthing folx can receive all of the services they need to have a safe and comfortable birth. The birth centre environment is suitable for families and children. Services are also organized to facilitate transfer to a hospital when needed.

A birth centre offers pros and cons that are similar to those of home birth. A major difference is the need to travel to the birth centre once in active labour. After delivery, the birthgiver and the newborn stay for about four hours before returning home. A midwife performs a home visit within 24 hours of birth and multiple visits over the following six weeks. They also provide infant feeding and baby care support.

In Hospital

Most pregnant people give birth in hospital, as most have either a family doctor or an OB/GYN as a healthcare provider. Many people perceive giving birth at a hospital as safer than in other settings because it comes with a large team of specialists, including anesthetists, obstetricians, pediatricians, and more. However, the number of interventions (including caesarean) is higher in hospitals for low-risk pregnancy candidates than in-home births (Association of Ontario Midwives, 2022a).

The Pros of Hospital Birth:

- Access to medication for pain relief, including epidural.
- Access to a large team of specialists.
- Access to operating room if caesarean is deemed necessary.
- Support from a labour and delivery nurse, even though their primary role is medical, and they devote a significant amount of their time to documentation.
- Possibility to add a doula to your support team (this option has not always been available during COVID-19 in most hospitals).

The Cons of Hospital Birth:

- Birthgiver must guess when they are in active labour to go to the hospital, which can result in multiple car rides while having contractions.
- May be harder to create an environment where the pregnant person feels safe and comfortable, and can relax, let go, and concentrate on labouring without disturbance.

- Increased likelihood of unwanted interventions, such as continuous fetal electronic monitoring, which limits mobility, blood pressure and temperature monitoring, regular (and painful) cervical exams, IV, augmentation, induction, and caesarean.

- Limited mobility due to continuous fetal monitoring during assessment at many hospitals.

- Less privacy due to the care personnel not being continuous, with nurses, doctors, and medical students (in teaching hospitals) providing care for a limited time and then leaving to care for others or shift change.

- Not all hospitals offer an "aquadural" (being immersed in water) and few hospitals allow water birth.

- Not all hospitals are baby-friendly or have policies conducive to a good start with breast/chest feeding. Only 44 hospitals and healthcare organizations in Canada are baby-friendly (Breastfeeding Committee for Canada, 2020).

- Policies and protocols vary significantly between hospitals.

For those who have a choice, one's health, location, how they envision their experience of birth, how previous birth(s) happened, values and beliefs, and culture are all elements that will guide their choice of birth setting and healthcare providers. Since home birth is often thought to be unsafe, more emphasis must be placed on informing pregnant people about the safety of this option. This is particularly important as part of contextualizing the assumption that hospitals are the safest places to give birth, despite rising rates of cesarean section, which is still a major surgery with its own risks. This is despite the evidence saying otherwise. The World Health Organization found that "as countries increase their caesarean section rates up to 10%, maternal and neonatal mortality decrease. However, caesarean section rates higher than 10% are not associated with reductions in maternal and newborn mortality rates" (World Health Organization, 2021). Still, as previously noted, cesarean rates have continued to increase in Canada, from 18.7% in 1997 to **28.2%** in 2016, representing a 50.8% increase in the past 20 years (Gu et al., 2020).

The differences among healthcare providers are in their particular training and in the model of care that they provide. The bottom line is that if pregnant people feel heard and respected, they have probably chosen the healthcare provider that is right for them.

We hope that this short introduction about birth settings and healthcare providers help prepare you to ask the right questions and to be an informed, prepared, and active participant in all aspects of your birth experience.

Indigenous Birthing and Canada's Birth Evacuation Policy

by Karen Lawford

My name is Karen Lawford, and I am an Anishinaabe midwife from the Treaty 3 area, which is 55,000 square miles spanning the provinces of Ontario and Manitoba in Canada. My family's customary land use area is between Lac Seul First Nation and Pikangikum First Nation. My family has lived in a remote way of being since time before time. Like her mother and her mother's mother, my mother was born on the land, but I was not born on the land. I am the first generation to not be born on the land.

My grandmother, my *kookum*, was also a midwife. I think her role was out of necessity because our people needed someone to learn how to deliver babies, so she became a caregiver. Knowing the mechanics of pregnancy, labour, and birth, as well as the related medicines allowed us to thrive. In contemporary times, we are fortunate that it is not often we think about things like surviving childbirth. I am so thankful for those caregivers who have dedicated their lives to doing this work. While I offer this gratitude, I also acknowledge there are people who have had horrible experiences with some caregivers, and some of these caregivers are midwives. We all have work to do as care providers to properly provide services to people who come to us for care. As an academic, my area of research is related to maternity care for those who live on reserves with a focus on Health Canada's evacuation policy. This federal policy requires people who live on reserves and are pregnant to travel outside of their community late in their pregnancy to birth in southern, urban tertiary care hospitals (Lawford, 2016).

Many Canadians have never heard of this policy and when they do learn of it, are surprised to know that it is still in effect. The evacuation policy for Indigenous Peoples is a direct action of colonialism and white supremacy, which are the main drivers in terms of assimilating and civilizing

Indigenous Peoples into a generic Canadian body politic. While the creation of this policy and those like it may have been built long before many of us were born, their devastating impacts continue to be felt by Indigenous Peoples today. It is within our collective power to change that.

When Canada was formed in 1867, the federal government committed acts of genocide via the Indian Residential School system, nutrition experiments, forced and coerced sterilization, the 60s Scoop, and the ongoing millennial scoop, to name but a few (Choate et al., 2021; MacDonald et al., 2014; Mosby, 2013; Sinclair, 2016; Stote, 2015) My archival research clearly demonstrates that interfering with Indigenous Peoples' sexual and reproductive healthcare was intentional and unequivocally linked with national efforts to destroy Indigenous Peoples at the very beginning of life. Indigenous people who are evacuated for labour and birthing services are forced to leave their homes and communities. In most instances, there is no other option and there is no choice.

I want to share a short conversation I had with a physician who worked in a northern area of Ontario and was quite familiar with the evacuation policy. He proudly told me that he called the police because a pregnant person would not get on the plane to be evacuated out for birth. As a result of his call, the pregnant person was escorted onto the plane in handcuffs, an intervention that some healthcare providers think is appropriate. I was astounded, a feeling that has since morphed into rage with a system that supports any care provider invoking the carceral state to remove Indigenous Peoples from their homes, communities, and lands. There is a severe and glaring disconnect between where care is provided and where people *want* to have their care provided. Indigenous people want to give birth in their home, in their communities, and with their families, just like everyone else. Of course, there are some people who do want to and need to travel for birth. It is the routineness and blanket application of the evacuation policy that is harming us all.

As a result of the evacuation policy, the number of healthcare providers who can deliver babies is decreasing because rural and remote maternity care units are being closed. This issue, which is often referred to as

Canada's maternity care crisis, is not just an issue for Indigenous Peoples but for all Canadians. The relocation of labour and birthing services to higher level hospitals that are located very close to the Canada/USA border is not only affecting Indigenous Peoples; it affects all Canadians. Consider, for example, the closure of the maternity care unit at the Stanton Hospital in Yellowknife, Northwest Territories. Between December 10th, 2021 and February 21st, 2022, everyone who would normally give birth in Yellowknife was forced to travel to Edmonton to give birth, which is almost 1,500 kilometers south.

This pre-emptive closure put birthing people at higher risk and created more stress because it also ended up happening during the COVID-19 pandemic. We must pay attention to where maternity care is provided, who provides it, and how we want it provided. Right now, Indigenous Peoples are not part of that decision making, nor are pregnant people. Instead, there seems to be a bureaucratic and administration lethargy that continues and is even widening the breadth of the Government of Canada's evacuation policy.

We must come to terms with the information I share because it is integral to the health and wellness of Indigenous Peoples and is affecting the way that maternity care is provided to Indigenous Peoples and to Canadians. The lack of care and the lack of choice in maternity care is unacceptable. We know that maternity care saves people's lives. We know there is a certain minimum standard of prenatal visits and postpartum visits, and who should be at a birth and the minimum training for that caregiver. I understand that some people choose to have unattended births because of the legitimate fears they have of encountering a healthcare system that seems to be losing its sense of humanity. I fear for our collective lack of humanity. The stories that are shared in this book are all relevant and serve as a reminder of our collective humanity. There is not one iconic birth story, but every story shared in this book has made an impact and has influenced how I view birth. I will end with one more story.

I remember that in midwifery school, we had a textbook describing people's experiences of birth. One of the pictures was of this woman; she was just hanging outside, and she was smoking. That's the reality. Some people smoke in pregnancy. Some people use substances that are not the best, but we need to support people without our own judgements clouding our ability to provide care in a good way. I hope that through reading the stories in this book so generously shared, we all feel listened to and inspired to unconditionally support the comprehensive, gender-inclusive sexual, and reproductive care that people want and so deserve.

Meegwetch

Editor's Note: Is this the first time you've heard of Canada's birth evacuation policy, which is still in action as of 2023? Do you want to learn more about it, and help contribute to changing this policy? We encourage you to look up more information by searching terms such as Canada's birth evacuation policy, forced evacuation of pregnant Indigenous women, and Canada's forced birth travel. To take action, you could write to your local government officials and let them know that you are against the birth evacuation policy and support investing in Indigenous and remote maternity care units. You could reach out to your local Indigenous maternity/birth group(s) and find out if there is other action being taken that you can contribute to. You can also read about the re-matriation of birth in the Nunavik province in northern Quebec in Daviss (1997), Houd (n.d.), and Epoo et al. (2021). After learning a bit more about how the Inuit of Nunavik have brought birth back home to their native villages and about the success of their model, you can advocate alongside and support other Indigenous groups doing the same.

Birthing as a Racialized Person: What Everyone Should Know

by Chandra Martini

What is it to be a racialized birthing person in this place and time? Sitting down to write something about this story, I lay out in front of me fragments of data, intuition, and memory. Small, exploratory studies. Extrapolations. Memories of the things overheard in hospitals, things I hoped the woman digging deep to bring her baby into the world was too engrossed to hear. Casual conversations with friends, midwives, doctors, nurses, clients, cousins. A consciousness of the diversity of BIPOC (Black, Indigenous, and people of colour) communities in Canada and the multiplicity of ways in which BIPOC birthing people and our families make sense of ourselves, our births, and our perinatal care.

The other day I had a conversation with my cousin Ashley and her husband Ike about their experience birthing their first baby. When their daughter LaRaeya was born just under the threshold for small for gestational age (SGA) according to the standard birth weight chart used in Calgary hospitals, they were told that they would need to keep her in the hospital for 36 hours for blood sugar monitoring per hospital policy. However, Ashley and Ike knew from conversations with their midwife that the practice of comparing all babies to a universal birth weight chart is controversial. Many researchers argue for the use of customized birth weight charts that take ethnicity into consideration, pointing out that Black babies tend to be born smaller, and Black SGA babies are less likely to experience morbidities like NICU admission and need for ventilation (Glauser, 2018; Melamed et al., 2014). When they brought this up with their nurses, Ashley says, their concerns were dismissed; "It was like we were stupid." She remembered what a delicate matter it was for them to advocate to bring their baby home before the policy's 36 hours:

> It definitely did not feel like you had any decision-making power at all. ... I work for Children's Services too, so I know – we get those referrals from the hospital, like, "Oh, Mom wasn't listening, ... Mom didn't follow medical advice."

While she pushed back against this policy that she felt was not designed with her and her baby in mind, she worried about being stigmatized as noncompliant. As a racialized person, she worried about what the consequences of that stigma might be.

So, it felt good, says Ashley, to connect with other Black new parents who had similar experiences. Sharing stories, she says, helped her feel less like "the outlier or the crazy one... even the birth weight thing. A lot of my friends went through it." She put me in touch with one of these friends, Linda, who said that throughout her pregnancy with her first baby, she felt an added burden to advocate for herself in a system that she felt wasn't made for her. This is a particular feature of sharing pregnancy and birth stories among her Black friends. She says:

> There just seems to be a mutual understanding that maybe other people who don't have our experience take for granted, that you just have to be your own advocate, and anything that you hear from your doctors, you have to call people who you know that also went through it to be, like, "Hey, does this sound right? Is this your experience?"

Ghost Stories and Birth Outcomes in Racialized Communities

Ike describes this exchange of mutual validation and information as the community's "ghost stories." He talked about families across his network of friends from the African diaspora in both Canada and the United States comparing notes about their experiences of things like recurrent miscarriages, ovarian cysts, prenatal care, and babies' birth weights. He described how these ghost stories ultimately accrete into a foundation of knowledge about what to expect and what to be wary of in seeking care for fertility, pregnancy, and birth.

While I have anecdotal information about the birth and perinatal care experiences of BIPOC people rooted in my own experiences as a midwife, a mother, and a biracial woman in Canada, there are little Canada-specific published data to provide a big-picture perspective on birth outcomes in this country. The picture emerging in the United States, where the data collected around race are much more robust, is troubling. Birth outcomes are worse in racialized and Indigenous populations in the United States, particularly in Black populations (Alhusen, Bower, Epstein, & Sharps, 2016; Thompson & Sutter, 2020). Preterm birth and low birth weight[2] are more common in Black babies (March of Dimes, 2015), and the infant mortality rate for Black babies is almost double that of White babies (March of Dimes, 2015). The 2016-2018 maternal mortality rate for non-Hispanic Black people was 41.4 out of every 100,000; that is three times higher than that of non-Hispanic White people at 13.7 for every 100,000 (Centers for Disease Control and Prevention, 2022).

Researchers are attempting to identify the reasons for these discrepancies, which are likely complex and multifactorial. Emerging evidence suggests that racial discrimination contributes to these outcomes through multiple pathways, including barriers to employment, effects of institutionalized racism in accessing perinatal care, and inflammatory processes related to chronic stress (Alhusen et al., 2016).

While the causes of these disparities are still a matter of inquiry, it is clear that they cannot be attributed to ethnicity alone. For instance, outcomes are better among Hispanic and Black people born elsewhere than for those born in the United States, and they get worse with longer time spent living in the United States, and with subsequent generations (Dominguez et al., 2009). Therefore, American statistics point out the importance of paying

---

2 I want to make a distinction here between small for gestational age (SGA) and low birth weight (LBW). SGA refers to babies born under the bottom 10th percentile for their gestational age, and therefore, compares a given baby to a statistical set represented on a growth curve. The use of standardized versus customized birth weight charts is a matter of debate, as discussed above. LBW, on the other hand, is an absolute category that denotes any baby under 2500 g. LBW can be due to prematurity, growth restriction, or both, and is associated with higher infant mortality and poorer long-term outcomes (Cutland et al., 2017).

attention to racial disparities in birth outcomes, but they cannot simply be extrapolated into the Canadian context. This is a country with a different healthcare system, its own unique historical relationship to its communities of colour, and its own national narrative about race and racism.

Missing Data and the Pitfalls of "Colourblind"

Race is not recorded on the Canadian birth documents, and in most cases, not reported in Canadian health surveys, so researchers attempting to uncover whether and how race plays a role in the health outcomes of people in a Canadian context have had to get creative. In 2017, researchers published the first Canadian population-level analysis of the relationship between experiences of racialized discrimination and health outcomes, analyzing a one-time supplement to the 2013 Canadian Community Health Survey that looked at experiences of discrimination in the Canadian population (Siddiqi, Shahidi, Ramraj, & Williams). This supplement provided a rare opportunity, as the Canadian government does not routinely report data by racial group, instead lumping all non-Indigenous people of colour into the umbrella category of "visual minority."

Siddiqi et al.'s (2017) study shows how this lumping obscures important information about the experiences and needs of specific groups, finding that different racial groups reported very different discrimination profiles, with Black people reporting the highest rates of discrimination, followed by Indigenous people. Further, they found that after controlling for demographic and socioeconomic variables, the experience of racial discrimination was associated with higher rates of chronic disease.

Sheppard et al. (2017), noting patchy and inconsistent reporting on birth outcomes for Indigenous people due to a lack of identifiers on birth registrations, linked data from a 2004-2006 cohort of births from the Canadian Live Birth, Infant Death and Stillbirth Database with the 2006 Census (the most recent one with a long form questionnaire). In this way, they achieved an indirect dataset on birth outcomes for First Nations, Inuit, and Métis people on a national scale. They found higher rates of preterm birth, stillbirth, and large for gestational age babies in the Indigenous group, and that infant mortality rates were more than double in the Indigenous group than the non-Indigenous group. Using a similar method, McKinnon et al. (2016) found that the disparity in preterm birth rates between Black and White babies seen in the United States is also reflected in the Canadian population.

Stories are powerful. They make meaning out of experience, they structure and reinforce our memories, they shape what feels important in the present and what is desirable and possible in the future. Canada has its own national story about race, itself shaped as a kind of foil to the one in the United States. Whereas racism is understood as a perennial problem in our neighbor to the south, the official narrative I grew up with is that Canada is a place where race is only relevant in as much as it adds pleasing variation to the benign mosaic of the nation. How many times have I been proudly told by people that they "don't see colour?" This narrative is implicit in the absence of race in Canadian birth registrations, the paucity of data on how race interacts with birth outcomes in Canada, and the fact that research on perinatal care and perinatal experiences for racialized people in Canada is still in its infancy (Adhopia, 2021). It has been Canadian policy to take a "colourblind" approach to birth outcomes.

But sometimes it's important to see colour. Ashley and Ike described the experience of their baby being tested for jaundice with a transcutaneous bilirubinometer, a tool that, even by their nurse's admission, doesn't work well for darker-skinned babies. They were getting readings well above the cutoff point at which babies need phototherapy and were preparing to have to admit him to hospital for this procedure before a more accurate blood sample was taken that showed his bilirubin levels would not require treatment. They were left wondering why they had gone through all that stress, why an instrument that doesn't work well for melanated babies was used on their melanated baby in the first place.

When I asked her whether she felt her Blackness was relevant to her perinatal care experience, Ashley talked about feeling like the system was playing catch-up to accommodate the needs and issues specific to her Blackness:

"The big piece is not having the statistics, and not having the equipment ... even like the jaundice thing, there needs to be a new standard of care that works for everybody." It's important for our healthcare system to see colour so that people of colour can feel seen.

Changing the System That "Wasn't Made For Us in the First Place"

In a system that does not make it a priority to understand the specific perinatal outcomes, experiences, and needs of BIPOC communities, disparities go unnoticed, and needs go unaddressed. Ashley describes it this way:

> The system just wasn't really built considering us ... the ovarian cyst thing as an example, it's way more common for Black women, and the doctors here, it's like they're playing catch-up almost. ... We just are blanketed with everybody else, but it's not really care for us.

Linda also articulated this frustration of seeking care in a system that "wasn't made for us in the first place," and for her, addressing this issue of invisibility starts with research in which race is made visible: "We need to go back to the drawing board and create evidence-based approaches and changes in how we're doing things based on what the data is showing now." We want to see these patterns that materialize out of the stories shared between friends and family tested against the scientific method and made actionable in publications that shape policy and practice. We want a healthcare system that acknowledges race, not to reinforce stereotypes, but to see and understand what disparities exist, address barriers and unconscious bias, and provide care that thoughtfully integrates the needs and concerns of BIPOC birthing people in Canada.

Stories have always shaped the way our perinatal care system works, or doesn't work, for those of us who encounter it. A narrative that frames race as irrelevant to the Canadian national identity has meant that to this point, it is difficult to get a clear picture of the birth outcomes and experiences of BIPOC people in Canada. Given the broader context of disturbing racial disparities seen in the United States and elsewhere, and emerging data suggesting similar disparities in Canada, it is long past time to make BIPOC birthing people visible in the way we report our data and in the research questions we are asking. In the absence of robust evidence of how and why race matters in fertility, pregnancy, birth, and parenting, we have our ghost stories. Our birth stories, the way we crosscheck and compare notes, the accounts of advocating for our babies and ourselves. These stories validate our experiences in a system that frames some of us as outliers, and eventually, as they accumulate, they become a signal to the system for how to do better.

Perinatal Care and Human Rights

by Lauren Miller

Do you remember completing puzzles as a child? Or perhaps, as an adult, you're still an avid jigsaw doer? Some puzzles line up smoothly, and the image looks seamless. Others don't quite fit into place, leaving raised edges, angled corners, and questions about the legitimacy of the puzzle, or whether the puzzle doer may need support in completing the puzzle.

The care provided to pregnant people is a lot like a puzzle. Ideally, it is a seamless match that flows as part of the larger journey towards becoming a parent (the first time, or again). Yes, sometimes it is seamless. But other times, the edges of the puzzle pieces are raised, corners are cut, and there are questions and concerns about the legitimacy of this care, as well as the need for additional support to ensure the patient is equipped with the necessary knowledge and skills to access the care that they have a right to.

This section explores the relationship between human rights and maternity care. Our goal is to help you ensure a seamless (metaphorical) puzzle for your/your patient's perinatal healthcare.

Adopted by the United Nations General Assembly in 1948, the Universal Declaration of Human Rights (UDHR) was created by people with different legal and cultural backgrounds from all regions of the world. For the first time in history, the UDHR provided a concrete, documented reference for the fundamental human rights to be universally protected. The Declaration is accessible around the world and holds the record as the most translated document in existence—over 500 languages! This work is our foundational guide to basic human rights.

> Everyone is entitled to all the rights and freedoms set forth in this Declaration, without distinction of any kind, such as race, colour, sex, language, religion, political or other opinion, national or social origin, property, birth or other status. - Article 2, UDHR (United Nations, 1948)

PERINATAL CARE AND HUMAN RIGHTS

Perinatal care—sometimes referred to as maternity care—is the healthcare and support a person receives while pregnant, during birth, and immediately after childbirth. Perinatal care can include a family doctor, obstetrician, midwife, doula, professional wellness (chiropractic, osteopathy, physiotherapy, etc.), and more. It is an umbrella term that covers a wide range of health and wellness services surrounding pregnancy.

There are direct relations between the UDHR and the perinatal healthcare system. Binding human rights and perinatal care into a successful system without disrespect or harm is imperative, and the right to equality, autonomy, and the use of law are a few elements of human rights that we examine here. Considering the transparency of social media, injustices are better documented now than ever before, and now is the time to better infuse perinatal care with human rights for all.

Situational Perspective and Human Rights

One's perspective has a lot to do with how one experiences perinatal care. Here we mean *situational* perspective, or the ways one's perspective is influenced by contextual factors, such as place (e.g., hospital or home), time (e.g., current day or 50 years ago), and one's role (e.g., obstetrician or patient). For example, an obstetrician and a birthing person who are both focused on the healthiest physical outcome for the birthing person and baby may not have the same situational perspective on how to go about this. Additionally, how each individual perceives actions, words, and behaviours differs from the next. If an obstetrician presents a recommended procedure in a manner of urgency to a patient, they may do so assuming the patient knows their right to ask questions or refuse. However, the patient could experience this situation as a person of authority telling them what to do without giving them a choice. The interpersonal relationships that birthing people have during this impactful and vulnerable time, including interactions between the care provider and birthing person, are critical moments and can be the defining factor in the patient have a positive birth experience.

For example, a global survey on childbirth psychological trauma asked birthing women who had experienced trauma to "describe the birth trauma and what you found traumatizing" (Reed et al., 2017). The majority of responses cited care provider actions and interactions as their key point of trauma, namely that respondents felt as though "care providers prioritized their own agendas over the needs of the woman" (Reed et al., 2017). Another study examined the perceptions women held with regard to their experiences of childbirth through the lens of human rights (Solnes et al., 2016). The study, with 17 participants from both rural and urban areas in Tanzania, showed that many of the participants felt their rights were disrespected. It is important to note that in many contexts, including but certainly not limited to low and middle income countries, structural factors such as inadequate facilities, overworked staff, and limited resources can exacerbate the likelihood of human rights violations. In the study in Tanzania,

> women's experiences of maternal health services reflect several sub-standard care factors relating to violations of multiple human rights principles. Women were aware that substandard care was present and described a range of ways how the services could be delivered that would venerate human rights principles. Prominent themes included: "being treated well and equal," "being respected," and "being given the appropriate information and medical treatment" (Solnes, et al., 2016, p.1).

Unconscious Racial Bias and Human Rights

Unfortunately, a provider can also unintentionally violate a patient's human rights, even when resources are abundant. For instance, a U.S.-based study found that racial bias can negatively impact the assessment and treatment of Black people's pain (Hoffman et al., 2016). That is, due to unconscious and false beliefs that many white people hold about Black people's higher pain tolerance, health providers (particularly white providers) may inadvertently dismiss, delay, or even deny pain management and other needed medical treatment to Black pregnant people. The devastating consequences of unconscious bias, as well as more overt racial discrimination, has been documented in numerous cases in the United States. This includes professional tennis player Serena Williams' recollection of her health concerns dismissed the day after giving birth and nearly dying as a result (Lockhart, 2018), and the tragic and entirely preventable death of Amber Isaac in childbirth (Olumhense, 2020), to name a few. The key takeaway here is that the human rights of people of colour, as well as gender nonbinary and transfolx, may be more vulnerable to being breached.

World Health Organization's Perinatal Human Rights

According to the World Health Organization (WHO), seven declared human rights correspond with perinatal care. Varying signs of disrespect diminish these rights. The WHO provides a breakdown of harmful actions and their corresponding rights:

Harmful Action	Human Right
Physical abuse	Freedom from harm and ill treatment
Non-consented care	Right to information, informed consent, and refusal, and respect for choices and preferences, including companionship during maternity care
Non-confidential care	Confidentiality, privacy
Non-dignified care (including verbal abuse)	Dignity, respect
Discrimination based on specific attributes	Equality, freedom from discrimination, equitable care
Abandonment or denial of care	Right to timely healthcare and to the highest attainable level of health
Detention in facilities	Liberty, autonomy, self-determination, and freedom from coercion

The WHO has a document for medical professionals outlining specific standards to be met in order to increase the quality of perinatal and infant care within health facilities. This document works as a guide to upholding human rights and includes characteristics of quality of care defined as "safe, effective, timely, efficient, equitable, and people-centred" (World Health Organization, 2022).

The framework, as it relates to pregnant people, considered eight domains in quality care. The domains are split between provisions and experience and include evidence-based practices, emotional support, functional referral systems, and effective communication, among others. The outcome of this framework is healthcare that balances key practice coverage with people-centred outcomes.

A human rights approach in perinatal care goes above and beyond individual perceptions, with a focus on respecting all human rights in every situation. It is the responsibility of all healthcare professionals to respect and protect the human rights of their patients. Yet, even when health providers have the best of intentions, a patient may not feel that their human rights are being respected due to a need for more knowledge, skills, and/or support. For example, the way a healthcare provider presents risks/benefits can create bias and complicate a patient's ability to make informed decisions. This is why ensuring that both healthcare providers and patients are equipped with knowledge of the patient's rights and skills to effectively communicate with one another are key components of the human rights-centred perinatal care puzzle.

By ensuring that healthcare providers are well-trained in human rights-based care and, correspondingly, patients are informed and prepared to advocate for what is best for themselves and their families, the perinatal care puzzle can fit smoothly and seamlessly together and maximize healthy and positive birth experiences for all.

Supporting Success: How Birthing Practices May Affect Breastfeeding

by Dr. Jack Newman and Teresa Pitman of the International Breastfeeding Centre

Most parents want to breastfeed their babies but may not have the information to know that what happens during labour and birth may affect breastfeeding. It's true that many parents give birth with multiple interventions and still breastfeed successfully. It is also true, however, that these interventions can cause significant challenges. By learning more about this, solutions can be more effectively identified and birthing person and baby can be well-supported on their feeding journey.

Here are some of the ways that interventions can interfere with breastfeeding:

Epidural Analgesia

Epidurals are commonly used during labour and can affect breastfeeding in at least three ways.

1. Intravenous fluids

When an epidural is administered, intravenous fluid is also given to prevent a drop in blood pressure. If the epidural is given over many hours, this can add up to a significant amount of fluid. What happens to all this fluid? Well, some of it goes into the mother's system, and some goes into the baby. Studies have shown that the more fluid the mother receives, the more likely the baby is to lose at least 10% of his birth weight. That number is noteworthy, because in many hospitals, a 10% decrease from birth weight automatically means supplementation, usually by bottle. (This response to a 10% weight loss is rarely questioned, but there are many factors that should be considered.)

That's not the only effect of the IV fluids. When a mother has received large amounts of fluids during labour, birth, and after the birth, she often retains a lot of that fluid for several days. Not only are her hands and feet often swollen, but also her nipples and areolas will be swollen, firm, and tender as well, making it difficult for the baby to latch on well (or at all) and get milk from the breast. Besides, the baby not getting milk well, a poor latch often leads to sore nipples. The solution too often suggested is supplementation with formula given by bottles.

2. Medications

Multiple studies have found that the medications used in the epidural can have significant effects on the baby, making it more difficult for them to latch on to the breast and feed soon after birth. The effects depend on the particular drug used and the length of time the epidural is in place, but typically, a baby will not latch on or suckle when positioned at the breast. Sometimes, the baby will take the nipple into his mouth but not suck. A newborn baby can normally crawl to the breast on his own if placed on the mother's bare chest. If an epidural was given, the baby is unlikely to be able to do this.

3. Fever in the mother

When mothers receive epidurals, they often develop a fever, and the longer they have the epidural, the more likely they are to have a high temperature.

How does this affect breastfeeding? The treatment for the fever typically includes antibiotics for the mother and the baby, and the baby may be taken to the special care nursery. The mother may be advised not to feed the baby in case she has an infection that could be passed on to her newborn. Although, if she did have an infection, the baby would already be exposed and would be protected by breastfeeding.

Oxytocin (Pitocin)

Oxytocin is often given to either start labour or to speed up labour by strengthening contraction. Oxytocin is also an important hormone during breastfeeding: the baby's suckling at the breast causes the release of oxytocin, and the oxytocin encourages the mother's milk to "let down" and flow into the baby's mouth.

However, studies have found that after being given oxytocin during labour, the mothers don't respond in the same way when the baby is at the breast. They produce less oxytocin and may have difficulty transferring enough milk to the baby in the first days after birth. Research also shows that these early difficulties contribute to ongoing problems with breastfeeding and early weaning.

Caesarean Section

Although Caesarean sections are sometimes needed and can save the lives of parents and babies, they can affect breastfeeding. A caesarean section is *not* minor surgery and there can be complications, such as infection and pain.

The hospital staff may separate mother and baby, in order to give the mother more time to rest and recover from the surgery. While support and rest are important, the separation means the baby can't breastfeed frequently and may be given bottles of formula instead.

The mother may experience pain that makes it hard to find a comfortable position to feed the baby. One study found that nearly 80% of mothers who had caesarean sections were still experiencing significant pain two months after giving birth and 18% said pain persisted to six months postpartum.

If the mother does develop an infection, she may be separated from the baby. She may also be given antibiotics and be advised not to breastfeed in case the medication affects the baby (it rarely does, though).

The Problems Caused by Interventions

1. Baby Does Not Latch On

Perhaps because of one of the interventions described previously (or other interventions), many new babies will not latch on to the breast in the first hours or days after birth.

What can be done to help the non-latching baby?

1. Be patient.

2. Keep the mother and baby in skin-to-skin contact, as much as possible. Often, the baby lying on the mother's body will find the breast and latch on, sometimes without any help at all. A nurse or other qualified health professional should be with the mother and baby, as the mother and/or baby may be affected by medication.

3. If the baby has not latched on within a few hours, the mother should get help to express her milk and feed the baby with a spoon or open cup. Hand expression often works better than a pump before the milk increases on day 3 or 4.

4. The mother should get qualified, skilled help with latching the baby in hospital and after going home.

5. She can use breast compression to increase the flow of milk from the breast, which will encourage the baby to latch on and stay on.

6. Stay calm. Many babies will latch on when the milk flow increases.

7. After day 3 or 4, when the mother's milk supply has increased and the baby is still not latching, using a tube to feed the baby as it sucks on a parent's finger frequently works to prepare the baby to take the breast. Finger feeding need be done only a short time before trying the baby on the breast.

8. Using a feeding tube at the breast if the baby does latch can help to encourage the baby to keep feeding.

9. Some babies are willing to experiment with latching on if they were first fed a little bit of milk via finger feeding or cup feeding.

10. Trying to latch the baby on right after the baby wakes up or just as the baby is falling asleep sometimes works well.

11. Babies who are crying and screaming have difficulties latching on. Showing the mother how to calm the baby can help the baby to latch on.

12. Making sure the mother expresses her milk and builds up a good milk supply is a main determinant in whether the baby will latch on. More milk means faster flow, and faster flow means the baby is more likely to latch on.

2. Milk Production Falters

During pregnancy, the breasts prepare for making milk for the expected baby. New milk ducts and glands are formed, and the milk-making system gets into gear. In the first couple of days after birth, the milk that is produced is called colostrum; it's made in small amounts but has high levels of antibodies and other essential components.

Then, over the next few days, the milk volume begins to increase. How much it increases depends on how much milk is removed from the breast, typically by the baby breastfeeding.

When the mother and baby are separated, or the baby doesn't latch, or the mother's oxytocin is low because of oxytocin during labour, this means that less milk is removed, and the breasts get the message to cut back on milk production. If the baby is being fed with bottles instead, it can become even more difficult because the baby quickly learns to change their way of suckling to fit the bottle nipple and may have even more trouble latching onto the breast. The baby also finds that sucking on the bottle quickly yields milk while going to the breast gives slower flow.

What else can you do?

Get good, experienced help with breastfeeding as soon as possible.

Even if breastfeeding doesn't get off to a great start, good help and support can get it back on track in many cases. The three points to keep in mind:

- Feed the baby, ideally with the mother's expressed milk, and using a method that doesn't involve a bottle.

- Keep removing milk with hand expression or a pump if the baby isn't breastfeeding.

- Keep the mother and baby together as much as possible, ideally skin-to-skin.

- Be patient. As the effects of the birth medications and interventions wear off, it usually becomes much easier to get breastfeeding going well.

Recipe for a Satisfying Birth

by Josée Leduc

SATISFACTION

Waiting Time: More or less, 40 weeks

Prep Time: 2 to 72 hours

Yield: 1 or more little humans, one or two new parent(s), new siblings, cousin(s), grandparent(s) and great-grandparent(s).

Category: Human Being

Method: Unmedicated or Medicated

This is a recipe that has existed since time immemorial. Every day, pregnant folks everywhere on the planet experience this incredible event. Not only the physical side of birthing, but also, and maybe even more importantly, the emotional side. This process not only results in the birth of a baby or babies, but of parents, too. A birthgiver may not feel satisfied if the recipe is followed but some ingredients are missing.

INGREDIENTS

- An enormous dose of support
- A good amount of patience
- Many breaths (breath in, breath out)
- A fair supply of understanding and trust in the birth process
- One protected bubble
- A huge dose of the 3 Rs (rhythm, relaxation, ritual)
- A high degree of respect for birthgiver's experience
- A large number of comfort measures and/or medication
- An ample amount of skin-to-skin contact between mother and baby
- One large load of love

INSTRUCTIONS

As with any recipe, variations are abundant. When baking a cake, butter, flour, and sugar are needed, but the proportions may be different depending on the recipe. Extras may be added or omitted to respond to elevation differences, the day's temperature, what's in the cupboard, and, of course, to make each confection unique.

The same goes for birth. Some little ones are speedy, and their births require less patience. Some birthers prefer to use medication for relief and may need a smaller dose of the 3 Rs. Each birthing person must find the right proportions to suit their own taste. The proportions in the recipe above are based on my own personal preferences and the observations of others' satisfying experiences.

During pre-labour, the birther must be patient, as it can be a lengthy process and may have an irregular pattern. Continue with your daily activities as usual until it is not possible to do so anymore.

Contact your support team and have faith in your body. Practice breathing through contractions with your chosen support person or people. Rest at night, if possible, and move during the day. Take a bath or shower as desired, eat when hungry, and stay well hydrated.

Once in active labour (defined as starting at 6 cm of cervical dilation), stay in your protected bubble, breath in, breath out, and let your support team take care of everything else around you. Just concentrate on labouring. Remember the 3 Rs (rhythm, relaxation, ritual*), which may come instinctively. Trust your instincts and listen to your body; it is wise.

Complement the ingredients above with whatever comfort measures you choose, and use as needed. Don't forget to change positions regularly, and move when possible.

If using the medicated method, continue to change position regularly and get rest if you can.

Respect must be given generously throughout the process of labour and birth to address the needs of your body and soul. The only person responsible for making decisions about your body and your baby is you. You should have evidenced-based information in order to make informed decisions that align with your personality, culture, beliefs, and past experiences. Without this important ingredient, the recipe will not give the expected result of satisfaction. You may also enlist the help of your support person for this step. Ensure that they are well informed and understand your preferences ahead of time so they can advocate for you if the situation calls for it.

Love should be sprinkled all over this process and can take many forms, depending on you and your support people. No one should ever have to give birth alone. Feeling safe and loved promotes a generous flow of the hormones that help the birth process along.

The final step of this recipe is skin-to-skin contact with the baby. This should preferably happen with you, the birthing person, but can be with someone else if needed or desired. This contact promotes the baby's health (warmth) and sense of safety, a good breastfeeding start if that method of feeding is chosen, and strong bonding.

Note about some ingredients:

Bubble: A calm, safe, and private environment

3 Rs*: Rhythm, relaxation, ritual.

Love: Compassion and support are a necessity at every stage.

Respect: Every birthing person is different, but they all need respect. Only evidence-based information, shared-decision making, and informed consent can provide a feeling of being heard and respected, which is paramount in having a satisfying birth.

* The 3 R's approach to childbirth preparation was noted by Penny Simkin based on observations of labouring women and how they cope with pain and stress in labour. There are three characteristics common to birthing people who cope well:

1. They are able to relax during and/or between contractions.

2. The use of rhythm characterizes their coping style.

3. They find and use rituals, that is, the repeated use of personally meaningful rhythmic activities with every contraction.

(This is a short summary of Penny Simkin's words about the Three Rs on page 147 of *A Birth Partner*.)

International Childbirth Initiative: 12 Steps to Safe and Respectful MotherBaby-Family Maternity Care

The following has been adapted from the International Childbirth Initiative website with permission from the IMBCO Board.[3]

The International MotherBaby Childbirth Organization (IMBCO), together with the International Federation of Gynecology and Obstetrics (FIGO), developed a global initiative to provide evidence-based guidance and support for safe and respectful maternity care. **The *International Childbirth Initiative (ICI): 12 Steps to Safe and Respectful MotherBaby-Family Maternity Care*** provides 12 clear steps for implementing evidence-based maternity care worldwide, acknowledging the interaction between the MotherBaby dyad, the family, and the environment, as well as their interactions with healthcare providers and with healthcare systems.

The ICI also supports the implementation of the 12 steps in maternity care facilities large and small and self-initiated quality improvement mechanisms that can be used to monitor the process, effect, and engagement in safe and respectful maternity services.

The creators of the ICI believe (and we do too!) that implementation of the 12 Steps will lead to better health and wellness for mothers and their babies, with more positive birth experiences and a better start to life within an environment of strong emotional attachment. The ICI, which is currently being implemented in over 60 sites around the world (see Lalonde, 2023 for a list of those sites), with many more on the way, has been endorsed by health professionals' organizations, advocacy groups, and childbirth education organizations, and support is growing. In short, the ICI Foundational Principles and 12 Steps provide a clear template for optimal maternity care.

---

[3] We have no specific affiliation with the initiative; we are including it because we believe it has value to improving perinatal care.

How to Use This Tool

Healthcare centres who offer perinatal care can apply to implement the initiative on the ICI website (www.icichildbirth.org). Healthcare workers can also request information about the process. Individuals can bring the 12 Steps to appointments with their care providers to discuss their preferences and show their interest in having this initiative implemented in their healthcare centre. Other organizations can also bring this initiative to the administrations of their local healthcare systems and request its implementation.

Here we provide the summary version, but you can go to their website to find the full version for more information: https://icichildbirth.org/initiative/

Step 1. Treat every woman and newborn with compassion, respect and dignity, without physical, verbal, or emotional abuse, providing culturally safe and culturally sensitive care that respects the individual's customs, values, and rights to self–expression, informed choice, and privacy.

Step 2. Respect every woman's right to access and receive non-discriminatory and free (or at least affordable) care throughout the continuum of childbearing, with the understanding that under no circumstances can a woman or baby be refused care or detained after birth for lack of payment.

Step 3. Routinely provide MotherBaby-Family maternity care. Incorporate value- and partnership-based care grounded in evidence-based practice and driven by health needs and expectations, as well as by health outcomes and cost effectiveness.

Step 4. Acknowledge the mother's right to continuous support during labour and birth, and inform her of its benefits. Ensure that she receives such support from providers and companions of her choice.

Step 5. Offer non-pharmacological comfort and pain relief measures during labour as safe first options. If pharmacological pain relief options are available and requested, explain their benefits and risks.

Step 6. Provide evidence-based practices beneficial for the MotherBaby-Family throughout the entire childbearing continuum.

Step 7. Avoid potentially harmful procedures and practices that have insufficient evidence of benefit outweighing risk for routine or frequent use in normal pregnancy, labour, birth, and the postpartum and neonatal period.

Step 8. Implement measures that enhance wellness and prevent illness for the MotherBaby-Family, including good nutrition, clean water, sanitation, hygiene, family planning, disease, complications prevention, and pre- and postnatal education.

Step 9. Provide appropriate obstetric, neonatal, and emergency treatment when needed. Ensure that staff are trained in recognizing (potentially) dangerous conditions and complications and in providing effective treatment or stabilization, and have established links for consultation and a safe and effective referral system.

Step 10. Have a supportive human resource policy in place for recruitment and retention of dedicated staff, and ensure that staff are safe, secure, respected, and enabled to provide good quality, collaborative, personalized care to women and newborns in a positive working environment.

Step 11. Provide a continuum of collaborative care with all relevant healthcare providers, institutions, and organizations with established plans and logistics for communication, consultation, and referral between all levels of care.

Step 12. Promote breastfeeding and skin-to-skin contact, refer to the 10 Steps of the Baby-Friendly Hospital Initiative, and integrate into practice, training, and policies.

The International Childbirth Initiative: 12 Steps to Safe and Respectful Maternity Care are protected under copyright and reproduced with permission of the ICI Executive Committee. Originally published in Lalonde A, Herschderfer K, Pascali-Bonaro D, et al. The International Childbirth Initiative: 12 steps to safe and respectful MotherBaby–Family maternity care. *Int J Gynecol Obstet.* 2019 Jul 1;146(1):65–73.

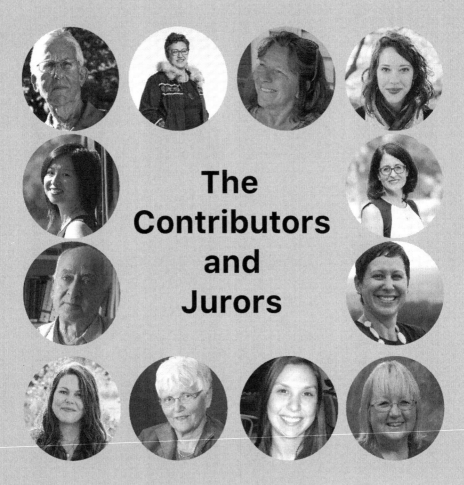

The Contributors and Jurors

About this collage: This is a collage of all those who contributed as jurors for the Birth Story Writing Contest or section writers to this book. We opted to share faces without attaching names in the hopes of representing the contributions to this book in the collaborative and collective effort in which they were experienced.

CONTRIBUTORS, CONTEST'S JURORS, AND ARTISTS

Book Contributors

Those who contributed their expertise to this book (other than the birth story writers) are listed here in alphabetical order.

Dr. Michael C. Klein

Foreword

Homage to Dr. Murray Enkin and the Complexity of Evidence-Based Medicine

Dr. Klein is the author of *Dissident Doctor: Catching Babies* and *Challenging the Medical Status Quo*. His early experiences working with midwives in Ethiopia were formative, leading him to question many standards but unjustified procedures in Western maternity healthcare. Dr. Klein is best known for his landmark randomized controlled trial of episiotomy, which demonstrated that routine episiotomy caused the very problems it was supposed to prevent. He played an important role in placing maternity care in the heart of family medicine. Dr. Klein kindly accepted to be on the Birth Story Writing Contest 2020 jury. The Doula Support Foundation was honoured to have him participate in the Birth Sharing Circle 2020 as well.

Karen Lawford

Indigenous Birthing and Canada's Birth Evacuation Policy

Karen is a Professor at Queen's University. Dr. Lawford is an Aboriginal midwife (Namegosibiing, Lac Seul First Nation, Treaty 3) and a registered Midwife (Ontario). Her research focuses on comprehensive, gender-inclusive sexual, and reproductive healthcare for Indigenous Peoples with a particular focus on the provision of maternity care for those who live on reserve. Karen kindly accepted to be on the Birth Story Writing Contest 2021 jury. The Doula Support Foundation was honoured to have her participate in the Birth Sharing Circle 2021 as well.

Josée Leduc

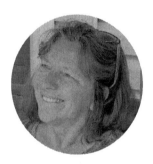

Introduction

Choosing a Healthcare Provider and Birth Setting

Recipe for a Satisfying Birth

Book co-editor

Josée, a birth doula CD(DONA) and French translator, is the creator of the Birth Story Writing Contest and Birth Sharing Circle. She is a DSF Board of Directors member. She felt the need for birth story sharing from her own clients, her own experiences, as well as the one from other doulas. Coming from the publishing world, she knows the power of words. She hopes that this book will contribute to a highly respectful birth environment everywhere and for all.

Chandra Martini

Birthing as a Racialized Person: What Everyone Should Know

Chandra Martini is a midwife and a descendant of the Black migration to Western Canada of 1910. She graduated from the Midwifery Program at Mount Royal University, where she worked with documents from the Black migration community to illuminate the history of Black midwives in Western Canada that had previously been eliminated from mainstream historical accounts.

Lauren Miller

Perinatal Care and Human Rights

Lauren Miller is a postpartum doula and educator with a history specializing in early childhood development. She has dabbled in freelance writing and enjoys any opportunity to combine the two. Lauren believes fiercely in the phrase "this too shall pass" as a humble guide for parenthood and a healthy reminder that the joyful moments pass just as the tough moments do. Lauren volunteers on the Board of Directors for DSF. She hopes that this collection of birth experiences gives a voice to birthers everywhere and shows the diversity and beauty found in birth.

Dr. Jack Newman

Supporting Success: How Birthing Practices May Affect Breastfeeding

Dr. Jack Newman is a world-renowned expert on breastfeeding. He founded the first hospital-based breastfeeding clinic in Canada in 1984, has been a consultant for UNICEF for the Baby Friendly Hospital Initiative, evaluating the first candidate hospitals in Gabon, the Ivory Coast and Canada, and founded the International Breastfeeding Centre in Toronto, where he and his staff provide care for over 2,500 mothers and babies a year. Dr. Newman has published numerous books, including a help guide for professionals and mothers on breastfeeding called *Dr. Jack Newman's Guide to Breastfeeding* (co-authored with Teresa Pitman) as well as *The Ultimate Breastfeeding Book of Answers*; *Breastfeeding: Empowering Parents* (co-authored with Andrea Polokova), and *What Doctors Don't Know about Breastfeeding* (co-authored with Andrea Polokova). His website www.ibconline.ca has information and video clips.

Laura Pascoe

Introduction

The Doula Support Foundation: A Short Story of our Birth

What is a Doula and How Can They Help Me?

Choosing a Healthcare Provider and Birth Setting

Book co-editor

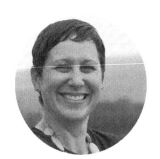

Laura Pascoe (M.S., PhD, CD) is a certified childbirth doula and co-founder of the Doula Support Foundation. In addition to her contributions to the birth and perinatal field, Laura works as an internationally experienced researcher, practitioner, and educator advancing evidence-based solutions to prevent violence and advance gender equality and sexual and reproductive health and rights. Her work primarily focuses on engaging and mobilizing men and boys as co-beneficiaries, stakeholders, and allies in creating a caring, just, healthy, and equal world for all. She lives in Vermont with her family.

Teresa Pitman

Supporting Success: How Birthing Practices May Affect Breastfeeding

Teresa Pitman has been a La Leche League Leader for more than 40 years. She is the author or co-author of 18 published books on birth, breastfeeding, parenting, and related topics, including *Dr. Jack Newman's Guide to Breastfeeding*, the 8th edition of *The Womanly Art of Breastfeeding*, *Preparing to Breastfeed: A Pregnant Woman's Guide*, and *Baby-Led Weaning*. She lives in Guelph, Ontario.

The Jurors of the 2019 and 2020 Birth Story Writing Contest

Bringing the jury together has been one of the wonders of the Birth Story Writing Contest. It brought people of different worlds together—the writing one and the perinatal one. Doctors, midwives, doulas, and writers read all the stories with so much respect and interest, which sparked thought-provoking conversation.

The jury for the first year's contest consisted of two Kingston writers and one of the first doulas who practiced in Kingston. Without their contributions, this book would not exist. The jury for the second year's contest consisted of two other local writers, one local midwife, and a family physician. Doulas and writers were also on the readers' committee to choose the longlist together. The experiences of working with these talented and thoughtful people generated wonderful and joyful connections.

Sarah Chisholm

Sarah is a registered midwife with Community Midwives of Kingston. Reading a variety of birth stories and being a doula are what ignited Sarah's passion for midwifery and client-centred care models. Bearing witness to the power of individuals during childbirth, made her passionate about obtaining skills that support people feeling safe and in charge during their childbearing experience. She is continually humbled by her work, and in awe of the individuals she works with.

Sue Cross

Sue is one of the first doulas in Kingston; she was a doula before most people in the area had heard of doulas. She has given a lot of her time supporting a large number of pregnant people in this area: people who could afford it, and people who could not. She has a generous heart.

Gretchen Huntley

Gretchen Huntley is an author from Kingston. She wrote three children's books, as well as a book on her son's journey with cancer. She is the founder of The Get-Well Gang, a group of crafters who make and donate 100% cotton caps to cancer patients. During the beginning of COVID-19, she turned to poetry to help her through the dark times. The outcome was a small poetry book called *Reality and Me*.

Michael C. Klein

Dr. Klein is the author of *Dissident Doctor: Catching Babies* and *Challenging the Medical Status Quo*. His early experiences working with midwives in Ethiopia were formative, leading him to question many standards but unjustified procedures in Western maternity healthcare. Dr. Klein is best known for his landmark RCT of episiotomy that demonstrated that routine episiotomy caused the very problems it was supposed to prevent. He played an important role in placing maternity care in the heart of family medicine.

Ying S. Lee

Y. S. Lee's fiction includes the critically acclaimed YA mystery series *The Agency*, which was translated into six languages and won the Canadian Children's Book Centre's inaugural John Spray Mystery Award. Ying's poems have been shortlisted for Australia's 2021 Peter Porter Poetry Prize, longlisted for the 2021 CBC Poetry Prize, and published in various journals. Her first picture book, *Mrs. Nobody*, will be published by Groundwood Books in 2024. Her website: www.yslee.com

Leanne Lieberman

Leanne Lieberman is the author of five young-adult novels, including *The Most Dangerous Thing, Gravity* (Sydney Taylor Notable), *The Book of Trees,* and *Lauren Yanofsky Hates the Holocaust* (Sydney Taylor Notable and Bank Street Best Book). Her latest book is just fresh from the press and titled *Cleaning Up*. Her adult fiction has been published in *New Quarterly, Descant, Fireweed, the Antigonish Review,* and *Grain*. Leanne lives and teaches in Kingston, Ontario. Her website: www.leanne.online

Lyn McCauley

Lyn McCauley joined this worthy collaboration with some experience in writing (a novel, *Early Release*) and playwriting (*Writing Romance*), and absolutely no experience in birthing or parenting. While it was not an entirely comfortable experience (understatement), Lyn was impressed by the creativity, humour, and courage displayed by the mothers who shared their unique and wonderful experiences.

Contributing Artists

These talented young artists kindly contributed the artwork found interspersed in the pages of this book. Jenn Grant is a wonderful musician who contributed her talent during the Birth Sharing Circle in 2020. We are incredibly grateful for their time, creativity, and talent they lent to making this book more joyful to engage with.

Mara Bureau

Mara Bureau is a young and emerging Canadian artist currently in her honours year in the BFA Program at Queens University. She primarily specializes in drawing, oil painting, and printmaking. Mara has worked as a fabrication assistant with various accomplished artists, and has exhibited her work at many galleries, including the Agnes Etherington Art Centre, the Union Gallery, and the Isabel Bader Centre.

Dominika Dembinski

Dominika Dembinski is an artist specializing in fine line work and oil painting. Her oeuvre focuses on the beauty of family, maternity, and industrial landscapes. She is an Art and English teacher and completed her Fine Art Bachelor of Honours and her Master's of Education at Queen's University. Her research focused on providing strategies for using arts-based interventions to mediate and therapize psycho-emotional distress in people's lives. She lives in Kingston, Ontario with her partner.

Jenn Grant

Jenn Grant was born on Prince Edward Island, the smallest province of Canada's maritimes. She's an award winning songwriter and performer, a painter, and a producer. The 3-time Juno nominee's music has been described by Australia's "The Age" as that of "dreamy, harp-and woodwinds folk, and the work of a painter born in paradise." She resides in Nova Scotia, where she is raising her two young sons alongside award-winning producer, husband, and long-time touring partner and collaborator, Daniel Ledwell. Beyond the borders of city life, art and music are being born every day. Jenn generously performed her song *Happy Birthday Baby!* to close the Birth Sharing Circle 2020, which was just perfect!

READING LIST

The quotes sprinkled through the book were taken from the favourite doulas' books of the Doula Support Foundation, and this list contains all of those plus a few extras! Most of those books are available at your local library or can be requested.

Babies are not pizzas: They are born not delivered, by Rebecca Dekker

Beyond Birth Plan, by Rhea Dempsey

Birth in Eight Cultures, edited by Robbie Davis-Floyd and Betty-Anne Daviss

Birthing from Within, by Pam England and Rob Horowitz

Birthing Models on the Human Rights Frontier: Speaking Truth to Power, edited by Betty-Anne Daviss & Robbie Davis-Floyd

Birthing with Confidence, by Rhea Dempsey

Birth Partner: A Complete Guide to Childbirth for Dads, Partners, Doulas, and All Other Labor Companions, by Penny Simkin

Birth: The Surprising History of How We are Born, by Tina Cassidy

Expecting Better, by Emily Oster

Ina May's Guide to Childbirth, by Ina May Gaskin

Like a Mother: A Feminist Journey Through the Science and Culture of Pregnancy, by Angela Garbes

Misconceptions by Naomi Wolf

Pregnancy After a Loss: A Guide to Pregnancy After a Miscarriage, Stillbirth, or Infant Death, by Carol Cirulli Lanham

Pregnancy, Childbirth and the Newborn – The Complete Guide, by Penny Simkin, Janet Whalley, Ann Keppler, Janelle Durham, and April Bolding

The Doula Book: How a Trained Labor Companion Can Help You Have a Shorter, Easier, and Healthier Birth, by Marshall H. Klaus, John H. Kennel, and Phyllis H. Klaus.

The First Forty Days: The Essential Art of Nourishing the New Mother, by Heng Ou, Amely Greeven, and Marisa Belger

The Happiest Baby on the Block: The New Way to Calm Crying and Help Your Newborn Baby Sleep Longer, by Harvey Karp

The Labor Progress Handbook, Early Interventions to Prevent and Treat Dystocia, by Penny Simkin, Lisa Hanson, Ruth Ancheta

TED Interviews podcast with Elizabeth Gilbert: https://www.themarginalian.org/2018/10/17/elizabeth-gilbert-ted-podcast-love-loss/

ACKNOWLEDGEMENTS

We often say that it takes a village to raise children. We would say it took a village to create this book. Creating this book opened up so many opportunities to meet great minds and hearts, and we humbly hope we give credit to all where credit is due.

First, I (Josée) would like to thank **Laura Pascoe,** former Chair of DSF, for believing and understanding where I was going with this project, and becoming a full-fledged participant by facilitating the **Birth Sharing Circle** with so much grace. It was an honour to work closely with this beautiful person on the book.

And I (Laura), offer my awe and appreciation for **Josée Leduc** who birthed this project and remained steadfast and endlessly creative throughout the planning and development of this book. Josée's generous, brave, resourceful, and kind way of being is easy for any who know her to see, and her leadership in breathing life and meaning into the Birth Story Writing Contest and all that's followed is truly inspirational. I am also deeply grateful for my partner and co-parent, John Haffner, for his endless love and support in all my endeavours, and my children for all they are and teach me.

And another massive and crowd-cheering thank you to all those who have and continue to make DSF run and provide doula support to those who most need it, including but not limited to Rachel Nafziger, Chelsea Loutsenko, Dina Day, Mandy McLellan, Bethany Geisel, Teaisha Whittingham, Anna Siwakoti, Lauren Miller, and Sophia Stickland. You are all incredible, and we are honoured to know you.

Then, in chronologic order of those who contributed directly to the Birth Story project, we would like to thank **Lyn McCauley**, a local writer from Kingston, Ontario. She made this contest possible by being one of the jurors. She brought along her friend, **Gretchen Huntley**, another local writer. You can also read one of her poems in this book. Then **Sue Cross**, one of the first doulas in Kingston, came along too. We will be grateful for ever to them to have been the very first jury of the DSF'S Birth Story Writing Contest. Thank you for your generosity, your involvement, and your honesty.

We have received every single birth story as a gift. Our deepest thanks go to **all participants** who sent their stories written from an honest and vulnerable place. I cannot emphasize enough the generosity of all **the 32 writers** who gave their story to this book. All royalties from this book will go towards giving doula support to those who could not otherwise afford them. Your generosity will allow birthers to have the support they need. We want to underline this gesture of solidarity.

For the second year of the Birth Story Writing Contest, **Dr. Michael C. Klein** graciously accepted the role of a juror and is such a huge support for birthing people and doula work in Canada. We are grateful for his enthusiasm for this project and were honoured that he wrote the foreword for this book. Thank you Dr. Klein for committing your career and beyond to improving perinatal care in Canada. We are also indebted to **Ying Lee** and **Leanne Lieberman**, two local authors who were on the 2020 jury. Your writer's point of view made this contest so rich. We were honoured to have **Sarah Chisholm**, a local midwife on the jury, and it means the world to us to have this collaboration and your invaluable, front-row-seat point of view too. I cannot underline enough their generosity in reading each received birth story with so much interest, heart, and intentionality. Thank you so much for your compassionate participation to the Birth Sharing Circle as well, and thank you for Dr. Karen Lawford for her powerful introduction for the 2021 Birth Sharing Circle.

Along the way we have met incredible contributors to add information we thought would complement the birth stories in meaningful ways. We are indebted to **Dr. Michael C. Klein, Dr. Karen Lawford, Chandra Martini, Teresa Pitman and Dr. Newman,** and DSF doula **Lauren Miller** for providing your time and expertise. Thank you for offering our readers concrete insight and guidance that can help them best prepare for caring for birthing people/birthgiving. To those who provided insightful edits and their incredibly generous reviews of this book—thank you for volunteering your time and voice to support this project.

To the many **perinatal organizations** that have helped making the contest known through social media, we thank you. The response from many writer's organizations has also been so welcoming and helpful. We are so very grateful that you spread the word. We want to mention the **Kingston and Frontenac Public Library** for sharing info about the contest and the Birth Sharing Circle on their social medias as well.

We'd like to also thank **Indigo Books & Music Inc.** in Kingston for letting us use their space for the first and pre-COVID Birth Sharing Circle. We are grateful to **Chelsea Loutsenko** for her support of this project and for gracefully helping us facilitate these very special events. We are in debt to **all the writers** who have shared their Birth Stories in the Circle. We also want to thank **all the jurors** who presented one of the writers during these fabulous circles. A million thanks to **Jenn Grant,** for listening to the Birth Sharing Circle and closing it with the perfect song: *Happy Birthday, Baby*. We are deeply grateful that Jenn brought her talent in such a generous way.

We would like to also acknowledge the time and value that **Stefanie Blackman**, a student in publishing, offered in the early stages of book planning and edited all of the birth stories. Her knack for making any text clearer and more concise has contributed immensely to this book.

Finally, we are indebted to Praeclarus Press for believing in this project, editing the manuscript professionally, making the ebook, and getting it all out to the world

We are amazed by the generosity, passion, solidarity, honesty, insights, integrity, enthusiasm, compassion and love that we have witnessed through this project.

With our deepest gratitude,

Josée and Laura

REFERENCES

Introduction

Alberta Midwives: Our Stories. (2020, November 12). Strong in her standing: One Black Alberta midwife shares her lineage, research and views. [Audio podcast episode]. In *Alberta Midwives: Our Stories*. Alberta Association of Midwives. https://www.alberta-midwives.ca/podcast/episode-02/strong-in-her-standing-one-black-alberta-midwife-shares-her-lineage-research-and-views

Ananda, K. M. (2011). Birthtellers: Healing birth through conscious storytelling. *Midwifery Today, 99*. https://www.midwiferytoday.com/mt-articles/birthtellers-healing-birth-conscious-storytelling/

Savage, J. S. (2001). Birth Stories: A way of knowing in childbirth education. *The Journal of Perinatal Education, 10*(2), 3–7. https://doi.org/10.1624/105812401X88138

Foreword

Enkin, M., Keirse, M.J.N.C., & Chalmers, I. (Eds). (1989). *Effective care in pregnancy and childbirth*. Oxford University Press.

Klein, M., Gauthier, R., Robbins, J., Kaczorowski, J., Jorgensen, S., Franco, E,. Johnson, B.,Waghorn, K., Gelfand, M., Guralnick, M., Luskey, G., & Joshi, J. (1994). Relation of episiotomy to perineal trauma and morbidity, sexual dysfunction and pelvic floor relaxation. *American Journal of Obstetrics and Gynecology, 171*(3), 591-8.

Klein, M.C,. Janssen, P.A., MacWilliams, L., Kaczorowski, J., & Johnson, B. (1997). Determinants of vaginal/perineal integrity and pelvic floor functioning in childbirth. *American Journal of Obstetrics and Gynecology, 76*(2), 403-10.

Klein, M.C. (2018). *Dissident doctor: Catching babies and challenging the medical status quo.* Douglas and McIntyre.

Enkin, M., Glouberman, S., & Jadad, A.J. (2006). Beyond evidence: The complexity of maternity care. *Birth 33*(4), 365-269.

Klein, M.C., Kaczorowski J., Robbins, J.M., Gauthier, R.J., Jorgensen, S.H., & Joshi, A.K. (1995). Physician beliefs and behaviour within a randomized controlled trial of episiotomy: consequences for women under their care. *Canadian Medical Association Journal, 153*(6), 769-779.

Klein, M.C. (1995). Studying episiotomy: When beliefs conflict with science. *Journal of Family Practice, 41*(5), 483-488.

Klein, M.C. (2009). A tribute to Phil Hall. *Birth, 36*(1), 4.

Klein, M. (1983). Contracting for trust in family practice obstetrics. *Canadian Family Physician,* 29, 22257.

The Doula Support Foundation: A Short Story of Our Birth

SisterSong. (2022, September 3). SisterSong. In *Wikipedia.* https://en.wikipedia.org/wiki/SisterSong

What is a Doula and How Can They Help Me?

Dekker, R. (2019). Evidence on: Doulas. *Evidence Based Birth.* https://evidencebasedbirth.com/the-evidence-for-doulas/

Dorward, L. (2018). We need more male doulas. *Vice.* https://www.vice.com/en/article/neqzp8/we-need-more-male-doulas

Dukehart, C. (2011). Doulas: Exploring a tradition of support. *NPR.* https://www.npr.org/sections/babyproject/2011/07/14/137827923/doulas-exploring-a-tradition-of-support

Gruber, K. J., Cupito, S. H., & Dobson, C. F. (2013). Impact of doulas on healthy birth outcomes. *The Journal of Perinatal Education*, *22*(1), 49–58. https://doi.org/10.1891/1058-1243.22.1.49

National Partnership for Women & Families. (2018). Continuous support for women duringcChildbirth: 2017 Cochrane review update key takeaways. *The Journal of Perinatal Education*, *27*(4), 193–197. https://doi.org/10.1891/1058-1243.27.4.193

Paynter, M., Matheson, L., McVicar, L., Jefferies, K., Gebre, K., Marshall, P., Thomas, L., Zylstra, G., MacEachern, D., & Palliser-Nicholas, F. (2022). Peer doula support training for Black and Indigenous groups in Nova Scotia, Canada: A community-based qualitative study. *Public Health Nursing*, *39*(1), 135–145. https://doi.org/10.1111/phn.12955

Vargas, R. B. (2021). Male doula helping men make birth process safer for Black moms. *Spectrum News 1*. https://spectrumnews1.com/ca/la-west/health/2021/06/08/male-doula-helping-birth-process-for-black-moms

Wodtke, L., Hayward, A., Nychuk, A., Doenmez, C., Sinclair, S., & Cidro, J. (2022). The need for sustainable funding for Indigenous doula services in Canada. *Women's Health*, *18*, 17455057221093928. https://doi.org/10.1177/17455057221093928

Choosing a Healthcare Provider and Birth Setting

Association of Ontario Midwives. (2022a). Home birth safety. *Home Birth Safety*. https://www.ontariomidwives.ca/home-birth-safety

Association of Ontario Midwives. (2022b, June 7). *#MidwiferyDataMatters: Examining the rise in out-of-hospital birth during the COVID-19 pandemic*. https://www.ontariomidwives.ca/midwiferydatamatters-examining-rise-out-hospital-birth-during-covid-19-pandemic

Breastfeeding Committee for Canada. (2020). *National BFI Quality Improvement Collaborative Project Participating Hospitals.* Breastfeeding Committee for Canada. https://breastfeedingcanada.ca/wp-content/uploads/2020/04/Hospital_Facility_List.pdf

Canadian Institute for Health Information. (2004). *Giving birth in Canada: Providers of maternity and infant care.* Canadian Institute for Health Information = Institut canadien d'information sur la santé. https://central.bac-lac.gc.ca/.item?id=providers&op=pdf&app=Library

Cheng, R. J., Fisher, A. C., & Nicholson, S. C. (2022). Interest in Home Birth During the COVID-19 Pandemic: Analysis of Google Trends Data. *Journal of Midwifery & Women's Health, 67*(4), 427–434. https://doi.org/10.1111/jmwh.13341

Cheyney, M., & Davis-Floyd, R. (2019). Birth as culturally marked and shaped. In R. Davis-Floyd & M. Cheyney (Eds.), *Birth in eight cultures* (pp. 1–16). Long Grove, IL: Waveland Press.

Daviss, B.-A., Anderson, D. A., & Johnson, K. C. (2021). Pivoting to Childbirth at Home or in Freestanding Birth Centers in the US During COVID-19: Safety, Economics and Logistics. *Frontiers in Sociology, 6.* https://www.frontiersin.org/articles/10.3389/fsoc.2021.618210

Goulem, B. (2022, January 17). KHSC announces new service providing midwifery support for newborns, parents. *The Kingston Whig Standard.* https://www.thewhig.com/news/local-news/khsc-announces-new-service-providing-midwifery-support-for-newborns-parents

Gu, J., Karmakar-Hore, S., Hogan, M.-E., Azzam, H. M., Barrett, J. F. R., Brown, A., Cook, J. L., Jain, V., Melamed, N., Smith, G. N., Zaltz, A., & Gurevich, Y. (2020). Examining Cesarean Section Rates in Canada Using the Modified Robson Classification. *Journal of Obstetrics and Gynaecology Canada, 42*(6), 757–765. https://doi.org/10.1016/j.jogc.2019.09.009

Hutton, E. K. (2016). The Safety of Home Birth. *Journal of Obstetrics and Gynaecology Canada, 38*(4), 331–333. https://doi.org/10.1016/j.jogc.2016.02.005

Jimenez, V., Klein, M. C., Hivon, M., & Mason, C. (2010). A mirage of change: Family-centered maternity care in practice. *Birth (Berkeley, Calif.), 37*(2), 160–167. https://doi.org/10.1111/j.1523-536X.2010.00396.x

Lawford, K. M., Giles, A. R., & Bourgeault, I. L. (2018). Canada's evacuation policy for pregnant First Nations women: Resignation, resilience, and resistance. *Women and Birth, 31*(6), 479–488. https://doi.org/10.1016/j.wombi.2018.01.009

MacDorman, M. F., Barnard-Mayers, R., & Declercq, E. (2022). United States community births increased by 20% from 2019 to 2020. *Birth (Berkeley, Calif.), 49*(3), 559–568. https://doi.org/10.1111/birt.12627

Malott, A. M., Kaufman, K., Thorpe, J., Saxell, L., Becker, G., Paulette, L., Ashe, A., Martin, K., Yeates, L., & Hutton, E. K. (2012). Models of Organization of Maternity Care by Midwives in Canada: A Descriptive Review. *Journal of Obstetrics and Gynaecology Canada, 34*(10), 961–970. https://doi.org/10.1016/S1701-2163(16)35411-1

Public Health Agency of Canada. (2020). *Chapter 3: Care during pregnancy*. Public Health Agency of Canada.

Simkin, P., Whalley, J., Keppler, A., Durham, J., & Bolding, A. (2018). *Pregnancy, childbirth, and the newborn: The complete guide* (5th ed.). Da Capo Lifelong Books. https://www.amazon.com/Pregnancy-Childbirth-Newborn-Complete-Guide/dp/0738284971

Vedam, S., Schummers, L., Stoll, K., Rogers, J., Klein, M. C., Fairbrother, N., Dharamsi, S., Liston, R., Chong, G. K., & Kaczorowski, J. (2012). The Canadian Birth Place Study: Describing maternity practice and providers' exposure to home birth. *Midwifery, 28*(5), 600–608. https://doi.org/10.1016/j.midw.2012.06.011

Vedam, S., Stoll, K., Schummers, L., Fairbrother, N., Klein, M. C., Thordarson, D., Kornelsen, J., Dharamsi, S., Rogers, J., Liston, R., & Kaczorowski, J. (2014). The Canadian birth place study: Examining maternity care provider attitudes and interprofessional conflict around planned home birth. *BMC Pregnancy and Childbirth, 14*(1), 353. https://doi.org/10.1186/1471-2393-14-353

World Health Organization (WHO). (2021, June 9). *WHO Statement on Caesarean Section Rates.* https://www.who.int/news-room/questions-and-answers/item/who-statement-on-caesarean-section-rates-frequently-asked-questions

Perinatal Care and Human Rights

Hoffman, K. M., Trawalter, S., Axt, J. R., & Oliver, M. N. (2016). Racial bias in pain assessment and treatment recommendations, and false beliefs about biological differences between blacks and whites. *Proceedings of the National Academy of Sciences of the United States of America, 113*(16), 4296–4301. https://doi.org/10.1073/pnas.1516047113

Lockhart, P. H. (2018, January 11). What Serena Williams's scary childbirth story says about medical treatment of black women. *Vox.* https://www.vox.com/identities/2018/1/11/16879984/serena-williams-childbirth-scare-black-women

Reed, R., Sharman, R. ,& Inglis, C. (2017). Women's descriptions of childbirth trauma relating to care provider actions and interactions. *BMC Pregnancy Childbirth, 17*(21). https://doi.org/10.1186/s12884-016-1197-0

Solnes, A., Lambermon, F., Hamelink, C., & Meguid, T. (2016). Maternity care and Human Rights: What do women think? *BMC International Health and Human Rights, 16*(1): 17. https://doi.org/10.1186/s12914-016-0091-1

United Nations. (n.d.). *Universal Declaration of Human Rights.* United Nations. https://www.un.org/en/about-us/universal-declaration-of-human-rights#:~:text=Article%202,property%2C%20birth%20or%20other%20status.

World Health Organization. (2022). *Quality of care*. World Health Organization. https://www.who.int/health-topics/quality-of-care#tab=tab_1

Indigenous Birthing and Canada's Birth Evacuation Policy

Choate, P., Bear Chief, R., Lindstrom, D., & CrazyBull, B. (2021). Sustaining cultural genocide—A look at Indigenous children in non-Indigenous placement and the place of judicial decision making—A Canadian example. *Laws, 10*(3), 59. https://doi.org/10.3390/laws10030059

Daviss, B. (1997). Heeding warnings from the canary, the whale, and the Inuit: A framework for analyzing competing types of knowledge about childbirth. In R. Davis-Floyd & C. Sargent (Eds.), *Childbirth and authoritative knowledge: Cross-cultural perspectives* (pp. 441-473). Berkeley CA: UC Press.

Epoo, B., Moorehouse, K., Tayara, M., Stonier, J., & Daviss, B. (2021). 'To bring back birth is to bring back life': The Nunavik story. In B. Daviss & R. Davis-Floyd (Eds.), *Birthing models on the human rights frontier: Speaking truth to power* (pp. 75-109). Abingdon, Oxon: Routledge.

Houd, S. (2016). The outcome of perinatal care in Inukjuak, Nunavik, Canada 1998-2002. Birth International. https://birthinternational.com/the-outcome-of-perinatal-care-in-inukjuak-nunavik-canada-1998-2002/#:~:text=It%20was%20very%20important%20for%20the%20people%20in,transfer%20during%20birth.%20The%20results%20have%20been%20reassuring.

Lawford, K. (2016). Locating invisible policies: Health Canada's evacuation policy as a case study. *Atlantis: Critical Studies in Gender, Culture & Social Justice, 37,* 2(2), 147-160.

MacDonald, N.E., Stanwick, R., & Lynk, A. (2014). Canada's shameful history of nutrition research on residential school children: The need for strong medical ethics in Aboriginal health research. *Paediatrics Child Health, 19*(2), 64.

Mosby, I. (2013). Administering colonial science: Nutrition research and human biomedical experimentation in Aboriginal communities and residential schools, 1942-1952. *Social History, XLVI*(91), 615-642.

Sinclair, R. (2016). The Indigenous child removal system in Canada: An examination of legal decision-making and racial bias. *First Peoples Child & Family Review, 11*(2), 8-18.

Stote, K. (2015). *An act of genocide: Colonialism and the sterilization of Aboriginal women.* Fernwood Publishing

Birthing as a Racialized Person: What Everyone Should Know

Adhopia, V. (2021, June 23). Why doctors want Canada to collect better data on Black maternal health. *CBC*. Retrieved from https://www.cbc.ca/news/health/canada-black-maternal-health-1.6075277

Alhusen, J. L., Bower, K. M., Epstein, E., & Sharps, P. (2016). Racial discrimination and adverse birth outcomes: An integrative review. *Journal of Midwifery & Women's Health, 61*(6), 707–720. https://doi.org/10.1111/jmwh.12490

Centers for Disease Control and Prevention. (2022). Pregnancy mortality surveillance system. *Centers for Disease Control and Prevention.* https://www.cdc.gov/reproductivehealth/maternal-mortality/pregnancy-mortality-surveillance-system.htm?CDC_AA_refVal=https%3A%2F%2Fwww.cdc.gov%2Freproductivehealth%2Fmaternalinfanthealth%2Fpregnancy-mortality-surveillance-system.htm

Cutland, C. L., Lackritz, E. M., Mallett-Moore, T., Bardají, A., Chandrasekaran, R., Lahariya, … Brighton Collaboration Low Birth Weight Working Group (2017). Low birth weight: Case definition & guidelines for data collection, analysis, and presentation of maternal immunization safety data. *Vaccine, 35*(48 Pt A), 6492–6500. https://doi.org/10.1016/j.vaccine.2017.01.049

Dominguez, T. P., Strong, E. F., Krieger, N., Gillman, M. W., & Rich-Edwards, J. W. (2009). Differences in the self-reported racism experiences of US-born and foreign-born Black pregnant women. *Social Science & Medicine*, 69(2), 258–265. https://doi.org/10.1016/j.socscimed.2009.03.022

Glauser, W. (2018). Ethnicity-based fetal growth charts could reduce inductions and elective caesarean sections. *CMAJ : Canadian Medical Association Journal, 190*(45), E1343–E1344. https://doi.org/10.1503/cmaj.109-5670

March of Dimes. (2015). Racial and ethnic disparities in birth outcomes. *March of Dimes.* https://www.marchofdimes.org/materials/March-of-Dimes-Racial-and-Ethnic-Disparities_feb-27-2015.pdf

McKinnon, B., Yang, S., Kramer, M. S., Bushnik, T., Sheppard, A. J., & Kaufman, J. S. (2016). Comparisons of black-white disparities in preterm birth between Canada and the United States. *CMAJ: Canadian Medical Association Journal, 188*(1), E19-E26.

Siddiqi, A., Shahidi, F., Ramraj, C., & Williams, D. (2017). Associations between race, discrimination and risk for chronic disease in a population-based sample from Canada. *Social Science & Medicine, 194*, 135–141. https://doi.org/10.1016/j.socscimed.2017.10.009

Sheppard, A., Shapiro, G. D., Bushnik, T., Wilkins, R., Perry, S., Kaufman, J.S., Yang, S. (2017). Birth outcomes among First Nations, Inuit and Métis populations. *Statistics Canada.* https://www150.statcan.gc.ca/n1/pub/82-003-x/2017011/article/54886-eng.htm

Thompson, J.A., & Suter, M.A. (2020). Estimating racial health disparities among adverse birth outcomes as deviations from the population rates. *BMC Pregnancy Childbirth 20*, 155. https://doi.org/10.1186/s12884-020-2847-9

Supporting Success: How Birthing Practices May Affect Breastfeeding

Beilin, Y., Bodian, C. A., Weiser, J., Hossain, S., Arnold, I., Feierman, D. E., Martin, G., & Holzman, I. (2005). Effect of labor epidural analgesia with and without fentanyl on infant breast-feeding: a prospective, randomized, double-blind study. *Anesthesiology, 103*(6), 1211–1217.

Brimdyr, K., Cadwell, K., Widström, A. M., Svensson, K., Neumann, M., Hart, E. A., Harrington, S., & Phillips, R. (2015). The association between common labor drugs and suckling when skin-to-skin during the first hour after birth. *Birth, 42*(4), 319–328.

Chantry, C. J., Nommsen-Rivers, L. A., Peerson, J. M., Cohen, R. J., & Dewey, K. G. (2011). Excess weight loss in first-born breastfed newborns relates to maternal intrapartum fluid balance. *Pediatrics, 127*(1), e171–e179.

Declercq, E., Cunningham, D.K., Johnson, C., & Sakala, C. (2008), Mothers' reports of postpartum pain associated with vaginal and cesarean deliveries: Results of a national survey. *Birth, 35*, 16-24

Dozier, A. M., Howard, C. R., Brownell, E. A., Wissler, R. N., Glantz, J. C., Ternullo, S. R., Thevenet-Morrison, K. N., Childs, C. K., & Lawrence, R. A. (2013). Labor epidural anesthesia, obstetric factors and breastfeeding cessation. *Maternal and Child Health Journal, 17*(4), 689–698.

Gu, V., Feeley, N., Gold, I., Hayton, B., Robins, S., Mackinnon, A., Samuel, S., Carter, C. S., & Zelkowitz, P. (2016). Intrapartum synthetic oxytocin and its effects on maternal well-being at two months postpartum. *Birth, 43*(1), 28–35.

Jonas, W., Johansson, L. M., Nissen, E., Ejdebäck, M., Ransjö-Arvidson, A. B., & Uvnäs-Moberg, K. (2009). Effects of intrapartum oxytocin administration and epidural analgesia on the concentration of plasma oxytocin and prolactin, in response to suckling during the second day postpartum. *Breastfeeding medicine: The official Journal of the Academy of Breastfeeding Medicine, 4*(2), 71–82.

Lavessona, T., Kalén, K., & Olofsson, P. (2018). Fetal and maternal temperatures during labor and delivery: A prospective descriptive study. *Journal of Maternal-Fetal & Neonatal Medicine, 213*, 1533-41.

Lieberman, E., Lang, J. M., Frigoletto, F., Jr, Richardson, D. K., Ringer, S. A., & Cohen, A. (1997). Epidural analgesia, intrapartum fever, and neonatal sepsis evaluation. *Pediatrics, 99*(3), 415–419.

Moisés, E. C., de Barros Duarte, L., de Carvalho Cavalli, R., Lanchote, V. L., Duarte, G., & da Cunha, S. P. (2005). Pharmacokinetics and transplacental distribution of fentanyl in epidural anesthesia for normal pregnant women. *European Journal of Clinical Pharmacology, 61*(7), 517–522.

Noel-Weiss, J., Woodend, A. K., & Groll, D. L. (2011). Iatrogenic newborn weight loss: Knowledge translation using a study protocol for your maternity setting. *International Breastfeeding Journal, 6*(1), 10.

Ransjö-Arvidson, A. B., Matthiesen, A. S., Lilja, G., Nissen, E., Widström, A. M., & Uvnäs-Moberg, K. (2001). Maternal analgesia during labor disturbs newborn behavior: Effects on breastfeeding, temperature, and crying. *Birth, 28*(1), 5–12.

Segal S. (2010). Labor epidural analgesia and maternal fever, *Anesthesia and analgesia, 111*(6), 1467–1475.

Torvaldsen, S., Roberts, C. L., Simpson, J. M., Thompson, J. F., & Ellwood, D. A. (2006). Intrapartum epidural analgesia and breastfeeding: A prospective cohort study. *International Breastfeeding Journal, 1*, 24.

Wiklund, I., Norman, M., Uvnäs-Moberg, K., Ransjö-Arvidson, A. B., & Andolf, E. (2009). Epidural analgesia: Breast-feeding success and related factors. *Midwifery, 25*(2), e31–e38.

The 12 Steps to Safe and Respectful Mother-Baby-Family Maternity Care

Lalonde A, Herschderfer K, Pascali-Bonaro D, et al. The International Childbirth Initiative: 12 steps to safe and respectful MotherBaby–Family maternity care. *Int J Gynecol Obstet*. 2019 Jul 1;146(1):65–73.

See also their website: https://icichildbirth.org/

Manufactured by Amazon.ca
Bolton, ON